Yoga for Singing

Yoga for Singing

A Developmental Tool for Technique & Performance

JUDITH E. CARMAN

OXFORD
UNIVERSITY PRESS

OXFORD
UNIVERSITY PRESS

Oxford University Press, Inc., publishes works that further
Oxford University's objective of excellence
in research, scholarship, and education.

Oxford   New York
Auckland   Cape Town   Dar es Salaam   Hong Kong   Karachi
Kuala Lumpur   Madrid   Melbourne   Mexico City   Nairobi
New Delhi   Shanghai   Taipei   Toronto

With offices in
Argentina   Austria   Brazil   Chile   Czech Republic   France   Greece
Guatemala   Hungary   Italy   Japan   Poland   Portugal   Singapore
South Korea   Switzerland   Thailand   Turkey   Ukraine   Vietnam

Copyright © 2012 by Oxford University Press

Published by Oxford University Press, Inc.
198 Madison Avenue, New York, New York 10016
www.oup.com

Oxford is a registered trademark of Oxford University Press

Library of Congress Cataloging-in-Publication Data
Carman, Judith E.
  Yoga for singing : a developmental tool for technique & performance /
by Judith E. Carman.
    p. cm.
  Includes bibliographical references and index.
  ISBN 978-0-19-975940-8 (hardback) –ISBN 978-0-19-975941-5 (pbk.)
  1. Hatha yoga. 2. Singers–Health and hygiene. I. Title.
    RA781.7.C3595 2011
    613.7'046—dc22   2010052012

To all singers everywhere,
and to all those whose song is yet unsung.

Contents

Preface   xiii

Acknowledgements   xvii

About the Companion Web Site   xx

PART I: *Theory and Techniques*

1. Yoga and Singing: The Connections   3

    Definition of Yoga   3

    Connections between Yoga and Singing   4

    Specific Objectives   7

    Structure and Content   8

2. Yoga and Singing: The Body   10

    Connections   10

    The *Viniyoga* Approach   10

    The Muscles of Singing   12

    Āsanas Especially Useful to the Developing Singer   13

        General Instructions for Āsana Practice   14

    Āsanas for Each Area   112

        Postural Muscles   112

        Movement Muscles and Joints   113

    Breath Adaptations in *Āsana*   114

        Metrical Inhale/Exhale Coordinated with Repetition
            of Movement   114

        Use of Various Lengths of Inhale/Exhale   115

        Use of Krama (Segmenting the Breath)   115

Use of Ratio (Inhale/Suspend/Exhale/Suspend)   116

Sample Sequences for Breath Adaptations in *Āsana*   117

A Sequence for Various Lengths of Metrical
Breath Patterns Video demonstrations are of Warrior
and Supine Forward Bend only   117

A Sequence for Krama Video demonstrations are
for Mountain (a) and Kneeling Forward
Bend only   119

A Sequence for Ratio Video demonstration
for Warrior (a) only   120

Sound in Asana   121

Use of Vowel Sounds on Exhale in Repetition
of Movement   121

Use as a Learning Device or to Sharpen Attention
and Memory   122

Sample Sequences for Sound in *Āsana*   123

A Sequence for Humming, Vowel, and
Consonant Sounds   123

A Sequence for Learning or Memorizing   124

3. Yoga and Singing: The Breath   125

Connections   125

The Muscles of Breathing   126

Prāṇāyāma Practices for Breath Development
and Control   128

Inhalation/Exhalation   128

The Singer's Breath   130

Krama: Segmented Inhale and Exhale   130

Breath Threshold   131

Ratio: Working with the Breath in Four Parts   133

Bandhas   136

Techniques: The Use of Different "Valves"   137

Four Alternate Nostril Breathing Practices   138

Other Breath-Related Practices   142

Humming   142

Patterns and Songs   143

Humming Exercises   143

The Breath as a Focal Point   144

4. Yoga and Singing: The Mind   145

Connections   145

The Mind of a Singer   146

The Coordinator   146

The Instrument of Learning   147

The One-Pointed Mind   147

The Relaxed Mind   148

The Mind Trained for Performance   148

Concentration Practices   148

For Mental Focus   149

For Weakening and Letting Go of Old
Thought Habits   149

For Forming New Habits   150

For Setting a New Direction   150

5. Yoga and Singing: The Heart   152

Connections   152

The Heart of the Singer   152

Meditation   153

Meditation Practices   155

Focus on the Breath   155

Use of "So-hum" or Other Mantra   155

"Big Sky" (thoughts as passing clouds)   156

Flowing River (thoughts as boats)   156

"Big Mind" (expansion from individual
to edges of the universe)   157

Metta (loving kindness meditation)   157

Contemplative Prayer (use of breath, religious icon,
meaningful word or mental image as
point of focus)   158

6. Yoga and Singing: The Performer   159

Connections   159

The Whole Singer   159

Command of the Body   159
Command of the Breath   160
Command of the Mind   161
Communication with Heart and Soul   161
Command of Relaxation   161
Deep Relaxation Practices   162
Tension and Release   162
31 or 61 Points   162
Awareness of Light in the Body   163
A Shorter Point-to-Point Awareness Relaxation   163
Conclusion   163

PART II: *Practices for Various Needs*

Chart of *Āsanas* Especially Useful to the Developing Singer   167

Sequences for Specific Areas of the Body   175
A Sequence to Strengthen Feet, Legs, Knees,
and Ankles   175
A Sequence to Strengthen the Lower
Abdominal Muscles   178
A Sequence to Stretch and Strengthen the
Lower Back   181
A Sequence to Stretch and Strengthen the
Upper Back   183
A Sequence to Loosen and Strengthen the Neck
and Shoulders   185
A Sequence to Open and Strengthen the Hips   188
A Sequence for Balance   190
A Complete Basic Practice for Daily Use   193
I. Āsana   196
II. Prāṇāyāma   197
III. Concentration/Meditation   197
IV. Deep Relaxation   197
Short Practices for Specific Vocal Deficiencies   197
Posture and Alignment   198

Breath Control   210
Mental Focus   216
Presence in Singing   219
Performance Anxiety   221
Anxiety, Anger, and Depression   225
Short Practices for Specific Situations   228
Energy States   228
Travel and Performance   235
Weight Issues   237

Afterword   243

Appendix: For the Voice Teacher   245

Notes   273

Glossary   277

References   279

Sanskrit Pronunciation Guide   281

Index   283

Preface

MY FIRST BRIEF encounter with yoga was in 1974 when my sister introduced me to a few basic postures. Over the next decade, I noticed increasing references to the practice of yoga, and in 1983 I bought B. K. S. Iyengar's book *The Concise Light on Yoga* as a supplement to the yoga classes I took that year. This first American edition of Iyengar's work was an adaptation of the original *Light on Yoga* published in England in 1966 and contained the original front material from the earlier book. Both Iyengar's scholarly and enlightening essay, "What Is Yoga?" and the Foreword by violinist Yehudi Menuhin, who had practiced yoga for thirty years as a pupil of Iyengar, made a lasting impression, though it would be almost another decade before I committed to my own daily practice.

At my first yoga class at the Yoga Institute of Houston, teacher Lex Gillan, quoting Ram Dass, said, "Some people really want to practice yoga; some *want* to want to practice yoga; and some just want to *want to* want to practice yoga." As time went on, I sank into the third category and remained an uncommitted novice until the spring of 1992.

As with many people of a certain age, I hit one of life's proverbial walls: "Who and where am I, and what am I doing here?" Such questions are only answered on the inside. To go inside, one must find a way to focus inward, to be quiet, to be at rest, and to become acquainted with oneself at last. Lacking the resources for outside help with this process, I returned to the practice of yoga in *āsana* and meditation. The positive fruits of this practice began to appear in a year or so, and I became committed to my practice.

As time passed, I began to notice how many yoga practices were directly related to the art of singing, and as a voice teacher, I began to explore these connections. After some consideration, I decided to take yoga teacher training and design a yoga course for singers. In the fall of 1999 I took a teacher training intensive course from my original yoga teacher and then designed a six-week session of classes especially for singers based on that training and

Iyengar's book. I taught the course to my own voice students and was able to see the effects of the yoga classes in their private voice lessons. Subsequently I offered this course to other singers in Houston, Texas. The original course served as a basis for sessions with church choirs, university classes, and the Houston Grand Opera Studio as well as ongoing private classes for several years until I felt a need for more training.

After taking some classes in various styles of yoga, reading a number of yoga books, and researching various yoga teacher training programs, I chose the American Viniyoga Institute's 500-hour Teacher Training course taught by Gary and Mirka Kraftsow. Four two-week sessions gave me the tools I needed to refine my yoga teaching, conduct national workshops, and write this book. I realized from the very first day of the training that the *Viniyoga* approach is perfect for singers.

I now base my teaching in the yoga lineage that comes from T. Krishnamacharya through his son T. K. V. Desicachar, and Desicachar's American student Gary Kraftsow rather than the lineage coming through B. K. S. Iyengar; however, two quotations from *Light on Yoga* make a strong connection between yoga and singing. Iyengar's definition of yoga in his Preface is a model of clarity, and Menuhin's definition of the practice of yoga resonates with all musicians—especially with singers.

"Yoga is a timeless pragmatic science evolved over thousands of years dealing with the physical, moral, mental and spiritual well being of man as a whole."[1]

"The practice of yoga induces a primary sense of measure and proportion. Reduced to our own body, our first instrument, we learn to play it, drawing from it maximum resonance and harmony."[2]

The name Krishnamacharya looms large in modern yoga teaching. Born in 1888 and living until 1989, his life and work span almost the entire twentieth century. The yoga teachings of those who were his pupils dominate yoga teaching in the West today. Considered to be the father of modern postural yoga, he was the teacher of B. K. S. Iyengar, Pattabhi Jois, Srivatsa Ramaswami, Indra Devi, his son T. K. V. Desikachar, and senior student A. G. Mohan. From these master teachers and their students who became master teachers flow most of the main styles of yoga teaching in the world today.

There are approximately fifteen to twenty distinct schools of yoga currently found in the United States. All cultivate the body with some form of *haṭha* yoga (physical postures) as well as various other practices: *prāṇāyāma*, concentration/meditation, chanting, study of Patañjali's *Yoga Sutras,* and deep relaxation. Various schools emphasize various different approaches and aspects of the totality of yoga philosophy and practice. The following thumbnail sketches of yoga teaching styles show how many possibilities are available to all kinds of students.

In general, the teaching of physical postures can be static or dynamic or a combination of both. Classes can be physical postures and some form of breath training only or emphasize greater meditative content. Physical postures can be taught in strict progressive series designed for strength, flexibility, and balance, or constructed for each individual class or each individual person's need. The teaching can be developmental or therapeutic in nature. Classes can be structured for individuals with specific illnesses. Classes can be highly active or more restorative and relaxing, or the teaching can be directed more specifically toward a spiritual goal. With these general categories in mind, the following list contains most of the American schools and styles of yoga and a very brief indication of the emphasis of the teaching.[3]

Haṭha: refers generically to physical postures and breath training

Ananda: highly meditative with simple postures and affirmations

Anusara: a combination of Iyengar-based postures with attitude, alignment, and action all flowing from the heart

Ashtanga Vinyasa: vigorous, fast-paced sequential series of postures

Bikram: strenuous; twenty-six traditional *haṭha* poses in a strict and unvarying order practiced in a superheated room

Himalayan Institute: Raja yoga—classical yoga including all eight limbs of Patañjali's description in the *Yoga Sutras*

Integral Yoga: classic postures with meditation

Integrative Yoga Therapy: emphasis on wellness and medical conditions

Iyengar: emphasis on precise alignment of postures that are held for long periods to find the subtleties of each one; use of props

Jivamukti: highly meditative form of Ashtanga yoga

Kripalu: flowing movements; willful practice, willful surrender (long holding of postures); meditation in motion

Kuṇḍalinī: postures and intense breathing practices to awaken the energy at the base of the spine

Phoenix Rising: classical yoga plus modern mind-body psychology; one-on-one teaching

Power Yoga: challenging series of postures to create heat and energy flow

Sivananda: classical yoga postures and other practices aimed toward answering the question, "Who am I?"

Tibetan Yoga: the Five Rites; emphasis on meditation

Viniyoga: all elements of classical yoga; individual adaptation; both dynamic and static physical postures; designed for the individual

alone or in a class setting; both developmental and therapeutic
in nature

Vinyāsa krama: all the elements of classical yoga with emphasis on a
flowing style, *Sutra* study, and chanting

All of these styles of yoga offer benefits to the dedicated practitioner, and most can be adapted for the singer according to the principles set forth in this book. In fact, the photographs in this book show postures both in *Viniyoga* style (the male model) and a style influenced by the Iyengar approach. The principles of *Viniyoga* regarding Repetition and Stay in postures coordinated with a metrical breath that facilitates faster or slower movement are easy to adapt to most other styles of yoga. The principles of breath development and control, mental concentration, meditation, and deep relaxation are also common to many other styles of yoga. The presentation of this material in the context of the *Viniyoga* lineage reflects the experiences, training, and best judgment of this author as singer, voice teacher, yoga practitioner, and yoga teacher.

Acknowledgements

MY FIRST THANKS are to my sister Carolyn who introduced me to yoga almost forty years ago, thereby planting the seed that has grown into this book. To my voice student, Edward Gabrielsen, I am indebted for pointing me toward my first yoga teacher, Lex Gillan, who encouraged me after my first teacher training with him to pursue the idea of creating yoga classes especially designed for singers. I am also indebted to yoga teacher Stan Hafner for introducing me to the principles of *viniyoga* that became the foundation of my work with singers.

My profound thanks go to Gary Kraftsow, founder and senior teacher of the American Viniyoga Institute, for his clear and masterful teaching of all the facets of yoga that are presented in this book. His emphasis on the role of the breath in *āsana*, concentration, meditation, and relaxation, as well as in *prāṇāyāma* and chanting, enabled me to make the connections with singing that made this book possible.

I am indebted to those first participants in yoga classes for singers, many of whom were my own voice students, for graciously allowing me to experiment on them. Two of those participants were voice teachers at the University of Houston, Katherine Ciesinski and Isabelle Ganz, both of whom had prior yoga experience and who have supported and encouraged me consistently since that time. I am also indebted to Kenneth Woods, formerly of the University of Central Missouri voice faculty, and to Stella D. Roden of the UCM voice faculty for making possible the pilot project of a semester of yoga classes for voice majors at the university. Thanks also go to the National Association of Teachers of Singing for providing opportunities to conduct workshops and classes at national meetings.

I am extremely fortunate to have had the services of professional photographer and longtime friend, David J. Schmoll, who both shot and edited the photographic images that illustrate the yoga postures and sequences. In addition, I offer my gratitude to yoga teachers Danielle E. Croft and Stacy Worley, owners of the Natchez Yoga Studio (Natchez, MS), and to Stan Hafner, owner of Austin Yoga Shala (Austin, TX) for their expertise as yoga models and for their willingness to participate in this project. I also offer my thanks to Thomas M. Mitchell, Assistant Professor of Photography at the University of Central Missouri for his helpful preliminary advice on the technical aspects of editing photo images.

I am extremely fortunate to have had the collaboration of videographer S. Jason Cole, Assistant Professor, Department of Communication, University of Central Missouri. His expertise in taping and editing the demonstration video found on the Oxford Companion Website was invaluable. Many thanks, also, go to the two UCM voice faculty members, Dr. Stella D. Roden and A. Jacob Sentgeorge, and the four UCM voice students, Nathan Gearke, Kimberly Tackett, Krystal Thurm, and Noah Whitmore, who gave unstintingly of their time and talent to make the demonstration video. Mr. Sentgeorge did double duty by also creating the musical examples at the end of the video.

Writing any book involves the input of many people besides the author, and this book is no exception. From start to finish, I have had the invaluable input and support of Dr. Rita M. Resch, singer, voice teacher, scholar, and friend. For the many readings and proofings of the manuscript throughout the writing and publication process, I offer my deepest thanks. Thanks are also due to longtime yoga teacher Anita Fischer for her reading of the manuscript and her encouragement of the project and to Dr. Ruth Doyle, longtime yoga practitioner and friend for a final reading of the text. I am indebted to Nancy Chapdelaine, fellow *viniyoga* trainee and teacher, for her critical reading of the text and checking of all the yoga postures and sequences, and to Andrew Sugarman, chanting teacher for the AVI teacher training courses, for his help with Sanskrit pronunciation. My thanks also go to Susanna Finnell, Joni Shereda, and Brian McKenna, all proficient in yoga, for their response to the manuscript and encouragement of the project. To friends and former students Jacqueline Hamilton and Anne and Tom Shepard of Houston, I extend my eternal gratitude for their hospitality and support during the photo shoots in Houston.

No book is published without major input from the editors and staff of the publisher. I have been fortunate indeed to have the help of the excellent Executive Editor, Suzanne Ryan, who took an immediate interest in my topic from the first time I contacted her. Her editorial assistants, Madelyn Sutton and Caelyn Cobb, have been invaluable for their consistent communication of information and advice, and production editor Erica Woods Tucker has skillfully shepherded the book through its final stages of production. Music book editor Norman Hirschy has been consistently and cheerfully helpful in the arduous process of producing the video for the companion website. I am also grateful to the two reviewers of my original manuscript for their suggestions and encouragement.

To all of the people named above, I offer my profound thanks for believing in this book and helping bring it to fruition.

About the Companion Website

www.oup.com/us/yogaforsinging

THE COMPANION WEBSITE to this book contains video materials and illustrations. The video demonstrations by two voice faculty members, three voice majors, and one theater major at the University of Central Missouri (Warrensburg) present all of the postures from the numbered Main *Āsana* List in Chapter 2, three short sequences for various purposes, seven breathing practices, two short practices from Part II, and a short demonstration class. The humming exercises from Chapter 3 are illustrated in notation, scale numbers, and interval names.

The video material, marked in the text by this callout symbol ⊙, is for demonstration purposes only and is not intended to serve as a full practice guide. For complete details about the video presentations, click on "About the Video Materials" on the website.

Readers may access the companion website using username Music4 and password Book2497. Please note that these are case-sensitive.

PART I

Theory and Techniques

1

Yoga and Singing

THE CONNECTIONS

Yoga is like music.
The rhythm of the body,
the melody of the mind and
harmony of the soul
create the symphony of life.

—B. K. S. IYENGAR

Definition of Yoga

Yoga is a tool for change—physical, mental, and spiritual. It is not just a single tool, but a whole system of tools called "practices" that address every facet of the whole person. The singer, perhaps more than any other musician—or indeed any other profession—is called upon to use in a coordinated way every facet of his or her being in public performance. For this reason, the practice of classical yoga is a powerful set of tools to help develop the singer's technique and performance skills.

The word "yoga," from the Indo-European root *yuj* meaning "to yoke," has many definitions. Among them are three that T. K. V. Desikachar illuminates in his book, *The Heart of Yoga: Developing a Personal Practice*. All three have relevance to singing in many ways.[1]

- yoga as the movement from one point to a higher point [or one level to a higher level]
- yoga as the bringing together, the unifying of two [or more] things
- yoga as action with undivided, uninterrupted attention

The act of singing, especially of operatic singing, is highly complex, involving every human faculty, and yet it must seem effortless. The soul has an innate need to sing; the heart has something to express in the singing; the mind must learn both the music to be sung and the technical skills to sing it. In addition, the mind must understand the text, create a character, learn to act as that character, project meaning and emotion in that character's life, and manage a host of other facets of performance. Moreover, the mind is the agent that connects the desire to sing to its expression through the physical body. The primary connector between mind and body is the breath. The unifying thread that runs throughout the practice of yoga is the focus on the breath. The same can be said of the art of singing.

Connections between Yoga and Singing

The connections between yoga and singing are many and intimate. Both require control of a strong and flexible body developed for freedom and endurance. Both rest on the foundation of awareness, control, and use of the breath. Both demand mental concentration and the ability to coordinate mind and body. Both lead to the knowledge and expression of the soul. Both open the heart. They are natural partners.[2]

An exploration of these connections for singers of every age and level of training and experience shows how the application of yoga practices works in building vocal technique and grounding the art of performance. Every trained singer goes through many stages of learning the elements of the art of singing. It is an ongoing process from the first lessons on posture and breathing, through initial performance experiences and refining vocal technique, to the pinnacle of one's ability in public performance and the effort to maintain a high level of consistency for as long as health and the instrument permit. There are yoga practices that support the singer's development and maintenance in each of these phases.

Singers beginning their formal training—even if they are gifted, physically well coordinated, and have been singing all their lives—generally have to learn how to use their voices in complex music or in specific performance styles and situations. The "natural singer" who seems to do everything right by instinct is rare. Singers in their teens have bodies that are still developing, and there are varying physical conditions that may need to be addressed—or simply physical techniques taught—before a degree of stability and consistency can be achieved. Basic upper body strength is often lacking, especially in teenage girls (unless they are athletes who develop the upper body), and this lack can impact the use of the breath. Yoga offers numerous physical postures (*āsanas*) to strengthen the muscles of the upper back that keep the chest up and open. Breathing practices (*prāṇāyāma*) strengthen the muscles that expand the lower ribs and keep them out as the action of the abdominal muscles supports the use of the breath in the sung phrase.

Although most serious young singers have a deep desire to sing, they sometimes lack the powers of mental concentration needed to turn their desire into the singing of their dreams. Their lives are overflowing with various activities that often crowd out the time needed for practice. Yoga offers concentration techniques that train the mind to focus in a one-pointed manner on the task at hand, without inner or outer distractions. This ability contributes to the effective use of practice time.

Young singers sometimes have emotional blocks of varying kinds and for varying reasons, things that condition their thoughts, emotions, and behavior in ways that seriously compromise the ability to sing well in public. Yoga offers meditation techniques designed to help the mind let go of unwanted thoughts and feelings, weaken old thought patterns, and build healthy, positive responses to stress. Some young singers appear to have no nerves, but others are painfully timid about public performance. Most become overly tense at the very time that a relaxed mind is needed. Yoga offers relaxation techniques for both mind and body that allow the singer to perform with a sense of ease and confidence.

Singers who continue their studies in a university music school setting encounter increased demands and stresses. Their bodies are still not fully developed. The only difference between a high school senior and a university freshman is three short summer months. The same problems that are present in their singing in high school will be present in their singing as freshmen voice majors. Moreover, the distractions of university life, even for the most dedicated student, can easily lead to difficulties with singing, especially in the freshman year. Add to this the increased pressures of adjusting to a new voice teacher, the music major's typically heavy class schedule, and music ensemble participation, and the stage is set for the winnowing process.

We used to think of university days as carefree, but for today's student the stresses are enormous, and health often suffers. Yoga offers practices designed to address all these areas and to make life easier and more manageable and singing more joyful for the university voice major. In addition, yoga practices designed especially for the singer can speed the implementation of vocal technique taught in the private lesson by offering developmental practices in a non-singing class setting for posture and alignment, breathing technique, mental focus, relaxation under stress, and numerous other areas.

The rising young professional singer encounters difficulties and stresses that only increase as success is gained. Unless there is strong financial backing, the necessity of the day job is ever present. The stresses of auditions, competitions, travel, performances, and constant money worries (not to mention personal relationships) all take their toll. The singer is no longer in the developmental stage of vocal technique but now must use that technique. To this singer, yoga offers the various physical and mental practices of an ongoing personal daily practice that keeps body, energy, and mind in balance and good health. For the singer established in a professional career, there is no better way to keep life in all its parts in balance than a daily personal yoga practice. As the professional singer matures and approaches the final years of public performance, daily yoga practice keeps the body supple, the mind focused, and the immune system strong.

The ancient practice of yoga was always considered to be a lifelong practice, evolving its elements from the vigor of youth to the demands and duties of middle age to the more gentle needs of old age. As the art of singing involves the participation of all the facets of the singer, so yoga involves training and maintaining all the facets of the person throughout life. It is truly a natural complement to the practice of the art of singing.

Patañjali, a yogi and grammarian who lived in India sometime between 200 B.C.E. and 200 C.E. codified the philosophy and practices of yoga into the classic text *Yoga Sutras*. This book of aphorisms sets forth the "Eight Limbs" (*aṣṭāṅga*) of yoga as a complete system: *yama* (universal moral commandments concerning one's relationship to others), *niyama* (self-disciplines concerning the relationship to oneself), *āsana* (physical posture), *prāṇāyāma* (breath expansion and control), *pratyāhāra* (withdrawal of the mind from the senses and exterior objects), *dhāraṇā* (mental concentration), *dhyāna* (meditation), and *samādhi* (a super-conscious state arising from deep meditation in which the individual merges with the universal).

It is important to note that the committed practice of yoga rests on and begins with the acceptance of the first two limbs. These are *yama*, five principles of respectful behavior in all relationships: abstaining from violence, falsehood, theft, extreme behavior, and greed; and *niyama*, five principles of relationship to oneself: purity, contentment, self-discipline, study of scriptures, and worship of the Divine. These are the moral components referred to by master yoga teacher B. K. S. Iyengar in his definition of yoga quoted in the Preface to this book and in the epigraph at the head of this chapter. The person who practices yoga in good faith will have come to the practice with some or many of these qualities already operative. The practice itself will develop each one, over time, to its highest potential in the person practicing. All of the principles of Patañjali 's "Eight Limbs" of yoga, directly and indirectly, apply to the art of singing in various ways (see table 1.1).

Table 1.1 **Principles of Singing Addressed in Yoga Practices**

Singing	Yoga

The Instrument (The Whole Body)
  Posture and Alignment
  Strength and Flexibility
  Coordination
	Physical Postures (*Āsana*)

The Power Source (The Breath)	Breathing Practices (*Prāṇāyāma*)
The Vibrator (Vocal Folds) and the Resonator Tonal Focus and Breath Flow	Humming/Chanting (Vocalizing)
The Command Center (The Mind/Brain)	Concentration Practices (*Pratyāhāra* and *Dhārana*)
The Expressive Center (The Heart)	Meditation Practices (*Dhyāna* and *Samādhi*)
The Awareness Center (The Relaxed and Open Body/Mind)	Deep Relaxation Techniques

The practice of yoga will support the art of singing in many ways for singers of all levels of training and experience. Participation in yoga classes designed specifically for singers offers several advantages to the student singer, among which are building community without competition, encouraging the establishment of good practice habits, and developing a sense of ensemble for group musical performances. Establishing a personal yoga practice, no matter how simple, will reinforce the habit of individual singing practice. Even if the student does not continue either with vocal studies or yoga practice, the seed of a lifelong practice for good health will have been planted, as many adults return to something begun in earlier years but abandoned for various reasons.

Specific Objectives

Yoga practices can undergird and strengthen the singer's art by helping to meet the following objectives:

- The development of proper posture and alignment for singing as well as a strong and flexible body for the many demands of singing on stage

- The development of strength in the muscles of the breathing mechanism, length of breath span, and breath control needed for lyrical singing
- The development of a smooth flow of breath in a well-placed tone
- The development of a one-pointed mind to focus in the moment and on the task at hand
- The development of the ability to let go of old thought patterns, form new habits, and open the heart, all important elements in dealing with performance anxiety
- The development of techniques to relax mind and body under the stress of performance

Singers can reach these objectives more quickly by engaging the practice of yoga as a partner to the study of singing.

Structure and Content

Part I of this book is divided into chapters on the body, the breath, the mind, the heart, and the whole person (the performer) in the same order as the practices of classical Raja yoga are taught. This structure is intended to present the elements of yoga for singers in a progressive manner in much the same sequence as the voice teacher might work with a beginning student, introducing the various practices to progress from the outer physical elements to the inner mental and expressive elements through the connecting agent of the breath. This structure will also facilitate finding specific practices in each area of concern.

The content of each chapter includes a brief discussion of the connections between the yoga practices presented and the singing principles to which they apply, an overview of the physical, mental, or expressive elements to be addressed, and the yoga techniques and practices themselves. Since this is a manual for practical use, the reader will encounter repetition of definitions and instructions as they apply to different practices.

Part II contains practices for use by all singers. Included are a numbered chart of postures (āsanas) for quick reference, sequences for various areas of the body, a guide to a complete practice for daily use, short practices for specific vocal problems, short practices for specific situations, and a section on weight control.

Appendix: For the Voice Teacher contains two sections: (1) very short practices for specific problems for use in the private studio with students who have no access to a yoga class; and (2) introductions and outlines for two semesters of progressive lessons suitable for use in Yoga for Singers classes at the university level or in other appropriate settings.

A Glossary of Sanskrit Terms with International Phonetic Alphabet Transcriptions for pronunciation follows the Notes. A Sanskrit Pronunciation Guide follows the References that provide sources of research for this book as well as for further study. The Posture Index alphabetizes *āsanas* both by their English and Sanskrit names.

The level of difficulty of each individual posture in chapter 2 and of each practice, whether given as examples in chapters or recommended in part II, is indicated by the following icon scheme: ♦ = Beginning; ♦ ♦ = Intermediate; ♦ ♦ ♦ = Advanced. These indications facilitate choosing postures and practices to suit the needs and level of expertise of each individual.

2

Yoga and Singing

THE BODY

Both require control of a strong and flexible body developed for freedom and endurance.

Connections

Movement is inherent in music. It is the property of meter and rhythm and the life of melody and harmony. Like dance that combines the movement of the body with the movement of music, the physical movement of the musical performer is often an intrinsic part of music making, a visual expression of sound shapes. The quotation at the beginning of chapter 1 from Indian yoga master and teacher, B. K. S. Iyengar bears repeating: "Yoga is like music. The rhythm of the body, the melody of the mind and harmony of the soul create the symphony of life." It is these elements of rhythm, melody, and harmony connected by the central thread of the breath that are so much like singing.

With our increasingly technological and sedentary society comes a loss of connection to our bodies that are so obviously made for movement. The child who spends long periods of time at the computer or watching television is not developing either connection to or awareness of the joys of a body in well-coordinated motion. For the singer, whose body *is* the musical instrument, this lack of body awareness is a serious problem that impacts many facets of his or her art, especially if the singer is also carrying excess weight. There are time-tested approaches to solving this problem, including Body Mapping, the Alexander Technique, Feldenkreis, and yoga. The focus here is on how the practice of yoga increases awareness of the body as a whole and offers specific ways of refining the body as a musical instrument.

The *Viniyoga* Approach

The approach to yoga called *Viniyoga* is particularly well suited for singers because of the central elements of movement repetition and coordination

with the breath in variable metrical patterns. The word *viniyoga* comes from
the classic text of yoga philosophy and tradition, the *Yoga Sūtras* of Patañjali
and is found in chapter 3, verse 6, in reference to the necessity of mastering
one thing before proceeding to the next step in a process. As with all Sanskrit
words, *viniyoga* has several meanings: employing, using, applying, disposing,
abandoning. Ultimately its complete meaning is evolution—"adapting the
means to each stage, intelligent use of acquired capacities, and transmission
as an offering."[1] This definition could also be applied to singing. Bernard
Bouanchaud quotes Indian yoga master and teacher T. K. V. Desikachar in an
elaboration of the meaning of *viniyoga*: "The spirit of *viniyoga* is starting from
where one finds oneself. As everybody is different and changes from time to
time, there can be no common starting point, and ready-made answers are
useless. The present situation must be examined and the habitually established status must be reexamined."[2] This elaboration also applies to singing.
A hallmark of the *viniyoga* approach is the adaptation of yoga practices to individual needs. This becomes important in relation to the different needs of
each individual singer.

The central focus of *Viniyoga* is the primacy of the breath in every practice,
physical or mental. All physical postures (*āsanas*) are coordinated with and
measured by a metrical pattern of inhalation/exhalation. It is this metrical (as
opposed to simply rhythmic) quality of breathing patterns that is so beneficial
to the singer (or to any musician) because singing itself—indeed, almost all
music making—exists within a metrical framework. Therefore, a complementary practice that uses a metrical framework reinforces the stability of
meter for the singer.

In addition to practicing *āsanas* with various metrical breathing patterns,
the exhalation phase of the breath can be turned into vocal sound, thus linking
the movement of the body with the duration of vowel sounds, short sung
phrases, chants, vocalises, or successive phrases of a song as an aid to memorizing. The use of vowel—and in some cases consonant—sounds in *āsana* is
an excellent way to practice the unfamiliar sounds of various singing languages.

The breath is also closely related to the movement of the spine, and primary focus on spinal movement in the physical postures builds awareness of
the extension and flexibility of the spine in posture and movement. This
awareness is important to the singer in the initial stages of training as well as
to the singer on stage who must keep the torso open and the spine as extended
as possible while singing in many different physical positions.

The primary focus of the *Viniyoga* approach to *āsana* is function
rather than form. This characteristic is of great value to singers, for whom

motion—both physical and musical—is of paramount importance. A primary focus on form implies static postures in which it is difficult for a beginner not to "hold" both body and breath with unfamiliar muscular tension.

The goals of *āsana* in *Viniyoga,* in order of importance, are these:

- Stability: being well grounded in one's stance
- Function: the smooth working of muscles, tendons, ligaments, and joints
- Strength: optimal strength of the muscles of posture and movement
- Flexibility: the ability to move easily in any direction from any position
- Balance: the feeling of a well-balanced body, on two legs or one
- Form: the achievement of the proper alignment in all postures

In the *viniyoga* approach, all postures are learned and practiced with a combination of repetition and stay. One moves into and out of a posture a predetermined number of times with a particular metrical breathing pattern, warming muscles and joints and paying attention to the biomechanics of the pose before ending in the "stay" position. Repetition promotes circulation to the large skeletal muscles, as well as developing their strength and flexibility. Stay promotes physiological changes in the inner body and deepening concentration through awareness of the breath. During "stay," the person polishes form by consciously addressing alignment of the body. An additional benefit of "stay" to the singer is consciously experiencing the absence of motion—silence and stillness—also periodically inherent in music but too often experienced merely as counting beats of rest.

The Muscles of Singing

All of the characteristics of *Viniyoga* discussed above serve specific needs for the singer. The starting point for addressing the body of the singer is an overview of the muscles that function in the act of singing. Since the whole body is the singing instrument, the whole body must be conditioned to function optimally. The postural muscles begin at the very base of the body with the *feet and legs,* which must be strong for long periods of standing and for many different kinds of movement. Next in importance are the *muscles of the pelvic floor,* the *lower abdominal muscles,* and the *muscles of the lower back.* These muscles form a girdle of strength for the trunk and are the root of the breathing mechanism. Resting on top of the lower trunk muscles are the *muscles of the upper back* that keep the spine erect and the chest up. Above the upper back muscles lie the *muscles of the shoulders and neck* that carry the weight of the head. The uppermost muscles of singing are the *palatal muscles* that elevate the soft palate and provide space for the resonance of the voice.

The muscles and joints of movement are also important to singers. Again, the muscles of the *feet and legs* must be strong, and the *joints of the ankles and knees* must be flexible and smooth. The muscles, tendons, and ligaments that support and move the *hip joints* must be strong and flexible for moving in different directions. The muscles and tendons of the *arms and shoulders* must be strong and flexible for various kinds of movement and for lifting or carrying objects as a function of a character on stage, or for holding a microphone for long periods of time in nonclassical singing. The muscles of the *neck* must be flexible and aligned for turning the head in different directions. Even the muscles of the *eyes* are important to the singer who must be able to focus at all distances, especially to see the conductor. The *breathing muscles* and *muscles of phonation* are discussed in chapter 3.

Āsanas Especially Useful to the Developing Singer

The following list of *āsanas* contains fifty-six basic postures plus two other exercises that are especially useful for singers in the developmental stage and for an ongoing practice. Each listing contains the English name of the posture, the Sanskrit name (for those already familiar with yoga) with International Phonetic Alphabet Symbols for correct pronunciation, the relation to singing, the general difficulty level, a brief description of the classical form of the posture, adaptations for the *viniyoga* approach, detailed instructions for moving into and out of the posture, common mistakes, risks, and contraindications (circumstances in which the posture should not be attempted or, in some cases, done with caution). In addition, photographs with breathing pattern and direction of movement illustrate the posture. Postures in part II and in the appendix are drawn from and referenced to this numbered list. For those who have no yoga experience, learning and practicing these *āsanas* in the manner described below should be a safe and profitable practice. For those who already have yoga experience, learning and practicing the *viniyoga* approach will be an excellent way to adapt that experience more specifically to the needs of singing. In both cases, it is important to coordinate all movement with the breath pattern specified initially. Once the posture is comfortable, the breath patterns can be changed in various ways—slowing down motion, prolonging stay, or working directly on the breath through repetition and stay. There are many possibilities, and almost everything will relate to singing in some way.

A major point of the repetition phase of each posture is the relation of tempo and smoothness of physical motion to an imagined sung phrase. A long observed phenomenon is the relation of hand and arm movement to the quality of singing. If one considers the possible problems in singing a long spinning phrase without stressing the breath, it is useful to observe the arm movement in *āsana* repetition. It is likely that the movement of the arm will display the same problems that one encounters in the sung phrase. For example, if one tends to give too much breath at the beginning of a phrase, one may also move the arms too fast at the beginning of the posture. If one tends to stop the arm movement at some point, or reach the endpoint before the end of the breath count, chances are that the same thing will happen at the same point in a sung phrase. Since it is easier to see arm movement than to sense breath flow, this is a good visual tool to diagnose breath flow disturbances.

General Instructions for Āsana Practice

Some general instructions for *āsana* practice are in order.

Practice all the elements of yoga on an empty stomach.

- *Inhale* (IN) while *raising* the arms and/or *opening* the front of the body (any form of stretching the front of the body vertically, or horizontally with the arms)
- *Exhale* (EX) while *lowering* the arms and/or *closing* the front of the body (any form of bringing the chest and thighs toward each other, or bringing the arms together in front of the chest)
- Practice each posture with a 4, 6, or 8-count (at 1 count per second, metronome marking M.M. 60)
  - inhalation and exhalation, moving into and out of the posture at the speed of and for the duration of the count
- Think of the flow of the breath and motion of the body as being the flow of a musical phrase
- Repeat the posture the number of times necessary for your needs of the moment
- Stay in the posture the length of count or breaths for your needs of the moment
- Always exhale completely before beginning movement into the initial phase of a posture, which usually occurs on inhalation
- In *standing* postures
  - Begin standing erect, feet straight forward, arms at sides, spine extended (*Samasthiti*)
  - Then move into the appropriate stance for the posture

- To stabilize the sacrum and protect the lower back
  - *Always* initiate the movement into forward bending postures by contracting the lowest abdominal muscles
  - *Always* keep the lowest abdominal muscles contracted when lifting the torso back to vertical

A cautionary note is in order here. In *āsana* work, go only to the feeling of a good stretch. Do not stretch to a point of pain. If you feel any pain at all, even the tiniest pinprick, stop immediately and move to a different posture. Moderation is the key to safe stretching. "Playing the edges"—yoga talk for pushing right up to one's limits—is a competitive athletic pursuit that can lead to injury and is not necessary for reaping all the benefits of these practices. Regardless of the commercial presentation of postural yoga in the United States, yoga is not a competitive sport. The central focus of yoga philosophy and practice is not "What can I do?" but "Who am I?"

Numbered Āsana List by Categories

Level of Difficulty indicated by ♦ (Beginning), ♦♦ (Intermediate), or ♦♦♦ (Advanced)

Positions:

- Standing
- Kneeling
- Prone
- Supine
- Seated
- Inverted

Directions:

- Axial Extension
- Forward Bends
- Backward Bends
- Lateral Bends
- Twists
- Balances

Standing Postures

Axial Extension

♦ 1. Balanced Standing Posture ▶

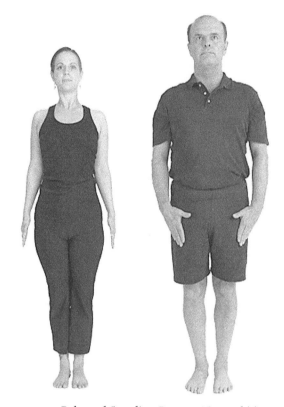

FIGURE 2.1 Balanced Standing Posture (*Samasthiti*)

Sanskrit Name: *Samasthiti* [sʌ mʌst ˈhɪ tɪ]
Category: Symmetrical Standing Balanced Posture
For the Singer: Identifies the balanced standing posture that is the basis of the balanced singing posture, the preparatory posture for all other standing postures
Difficulty Level: Beginning
Classic Form: Standing erect and still; feet together; arms at sides, palms facing thighs; spine extended; head in line with spine; back of neck lengthened; chin slightly down

Viniyoga **Adaptations:** Feet slightly apart
Instructions:

1) Stand with feet slightly apart, knees unlocked, toes aligned straight forward, arms at sides
2) Inhaling, lift the chest and expand the lower ribs and the abdominal muscles; lengthen the back of the neck by slightly tucking the chin
3) Exhaling, contract the abdominal muscles, keeping the chest up and expanded as long as possible; relax shoulders and arms
4) Take 4 breaths maintaining this posture

> **Common Mistakes:** Standing too rigidly; locking the knees, feet not parallel, feet too close together or too far apart
> **Risks:** None

♦ **2. Mountain Posture (with arm and heel raises) (a), (b), (c), (d), (e)** ▶

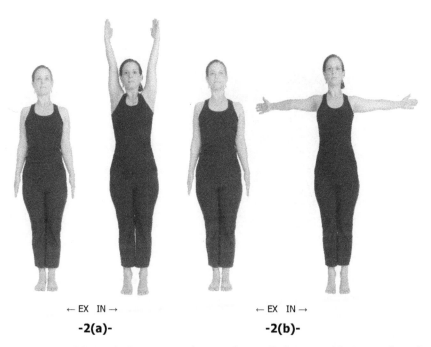

← EX   IN →   ← EX   IN →

-2(a)-   **-2(b)-**

FIGURE 2.2 Mountain Posture (a), (b), (c), (d), (e) (*Tāḍāsana*) with Arm and Heel Raises

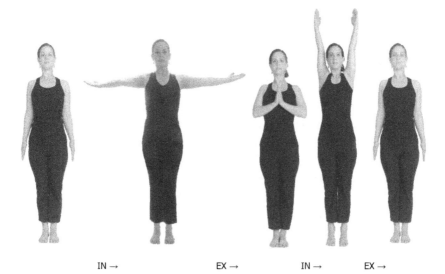

IN →   EX →   IN →   EX →

-2(c)-

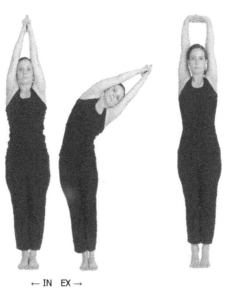

← IN   EX →

-2(d)-   **-2(e)-**

Sanskrit Name: *Tāḍāsana* [ta ˈda sʌ nʌ]

Category: Symmetrical Standing Axial Extension

For the Singer: Trains proper singing posture for the torso (feet and leg placement in singing may be different from the classic pose); extends the spine; opens the chest; strengthens feet and legs; improves balance

Difficulty Level: Beginning

Classic Form: An erect standing posture: feet together and toes straight forward with arches slightly lifted, spine erect, shoulder blades down and toward the spine, head slightly back in line with spine, chin very slightly down, shoulders down, arms relaxed, chest lifted; "Mountain" with arms raised straight overhead, fingers interlocked and rotated upward

***Viniyoga* Adaptations:** Include different placement of feet for structural reasons and use of arm and heel raises coordinated with the breath for movement in the posture

Instructions:

1) Stand in *Samasthiti* (see #1): exhale completely; coordinate length of breath (Inhale 4/Exhale 4 at metronome marking M.M. 60) with movement of arm and heel raises, as though each full breath and movement are in the context of two measures of 4/4 meter; repeat (a) and (b) 4 times, (c) twice, (d) twice; stay in (e) 3 breaths

2) Inhaling 4 counts, raise both arms forward and straight up beside ears, palms facing outward or toward each other, simultaneously lifting heels slightly off the floor (a)

3) Exhaling 4 counts, lower arms to sides

4) Inhaling 4 counts, bring arms forward, up, and out horizontally, palms facing upward (b)

5) Exhaling 4 counts, lower arms to sides

6) Inhaling 4 counts, bring arms out horizontally, palms facing upward (c)

7) Exhaling 4 counts, bring palms together at center of chest

8) Inhaling 4 counts, reach arms back and up straight overhead, lifting heels slightly off floor

9) Exhaling 4 counts, lower arms to sides and heels to floor

10) Inhaling 4 counts, raise arms straight overhead, clasp hands, elbows close to ears, heels on floor

11) Exhaling 4 counts, keeping hips in place and head in line with spine, bend to the right (d)

12) Inhaling 4 counts, return to center

13) Exhaling 4 counts, bend to the left

14) Inhaling 4 counts, return to center, turn clasped hands over and push toward ceiling, raising heels slightly off floor (e)

15) Exhaling 4 counts, lower backs of clasped hands to top of head

16) Inhaling 4 counts, push hands toward ceiling

17) Exhaling 4 counts, lower clasped hands to back of neck, pulling shoulder blades together and down the back

18) Inhaling 4 counts, push hands toward ceiling

19) Exhaling 4 counts, lower clasped hands forward, release hands to sides and heels to floor

> **Common Mistakes:** Include lifting the heels too high off the floor and balancing on toes instead of balls of feet; allowing feet to roll outward, causing a loss of balance; over-rotating the shoulders in the arm lifts; failing to contract abdominal muscles for stability of sacrum and balance
>
> **Risks:** overstretched shoulder muscles; loss of balance
>
> **Contraindications:** foot injury; dizziness; shoulder injury

FORWARD BENDS

♦ 3. Standing Forward Bend ▶

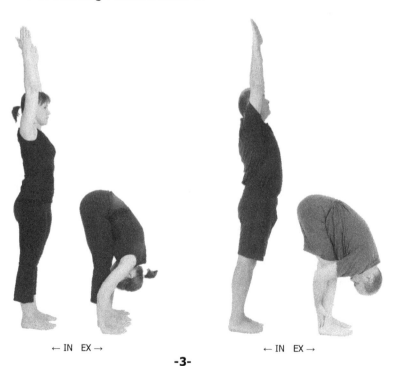

← IN EX →   ← IN EX →

-3-

FIGURE 2.3 Standing Forward Bend (*Uttānāsana*)

Sanskrit Name: *Uttānāsana* [ʊt: ta 'na sʌ nʌ]
Category: Symmetrical Standing Forward Bend
For the Singer: Provides a deep stretch of the spinal muscles
and strong work in the trunk flexors as well as the hamstrings,
quadriceps, and shoulder girdle in returning to the upright position;
abdominal muscles are strengthened by remaining contracted
throughout the movements of the posture
Difficulty Level: Beginning
Classic Form: Feet together, straight legs, chest on thighs, hands
flat on floor beside feet, head down
***Viniyoga* Adaptations:** Feet slightly apart; knees slightly bent to
release the hamstrings and protect the lower back; arm adaptations
Instructions:

1) Stand with feet slightly apart, knees unlocked, weight evenly distributed on
   feet, arches pulled up; exhale completely
2) Inhaling, lift chest away from belly and raise arms overhead
3) Exhaling, contract lower abdominal muscles to initiate forward bend,
   slightly bending knees, keeping head, chest, and arms aligned (or sweeping arms outward and down as in a swan dive, or running hands down
   backs of legs) and upper back as flat as possible (by pulling the shoulder
   blades together and down); bring hands to ankles or floor, release torso
   downward, tuck chin
4) Inhaling, abdominals contracted, pull chest and arms forward and up (or
   sweep arms behind and up), leading with the chest; keep upper back flat
   and weight firmly on heels; return to upright position
5) Exhaling, lower arms to sides

   Common Mistakes: Excessive forward rotation of pelvis;
   collapsing chest over belly; shifting weight to balls of feet; rotation
   of knees; collapsing arches; jutting chin forward
   Risks: Compression or strain in lower back; strain in neck and
   shoulders; accumulated tension
   Contraindications: Lower back or neck injuries; blood pressure
   issues

♦ ♦ 4. Standing Half Forward Bend ▶

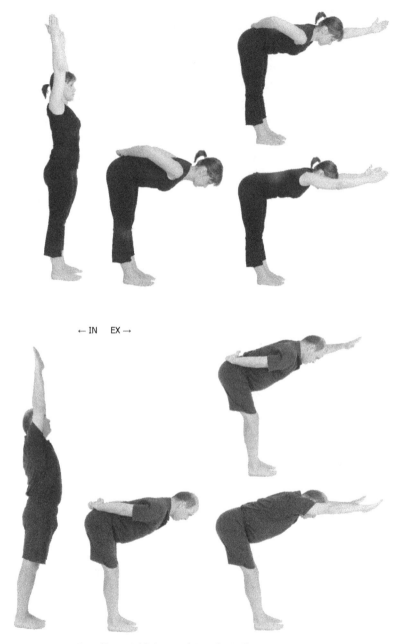

← IN   EX →

FIGURE 2.4   Standing Half Forward Bend (*Ardha Uttānāsana*)

Sanskrit Name: *Ardha Uttānāsana* [ˈʌrd hʌ - ʊtː ta ˈna sʌ nʌ]
Category: Symmetrical Standing Half Forward Bend
For the Singer: Builds strength in the lower abdominal muscles as they remain contracted throughout the movements of the posture; primary intention of the posture is to stretch and strengthen the musculature of the entire back
Difficulty Level: Intermediate
Classic Form: A variation of *Uttānāsana* in which torso and arms are lifted from the full forward bend and held parallel to the floor; legs together and straight; arms together and straight beside ears at right angle to legs; chin tucked in
Viniyoga **Adaptations:** Feet slightly apart; knees slightly bent to release hamstrings; one or both arms behind back to reduce workload on lower back
Instructions:

1) Stand with feet slightly apart, knees unlocked, weight evenly distributed on both feet, arches lifted; exhale completely
2) Inhaling, lift chest away from the belly and raise arms overhead
3) Exhaling, begin forward bend by contracting abdominals at pubis; keeping weight on heels, slightly bend knees while bending forward; keeping upper back as flat as possible, align head, arms, and chest; repeat 2–3 times and/ or continue into full forward bend and release weight of upper body, tucking chin slightly; abdominals remain contracted
4) Inhaling, keeping heels firmly on the floor and leading with the chest, pull chest and arms forward and up halfway, parallel to the floor; abdominals remain contracted and upper back flat
5) Exhaling, contract abdominals and remain in position, or return to full forward bend
6) Inhaling, return to halfway position or to full upright position
7) Exhaling, lower arms to sides

Common Mistakes: Excessive forward rotation of pelvis; collapsing chest over belly; shifting weight to balls of feet; rotation of knees; collapsing arches; jutting chin forward
Risks: Compression or strain in lower back; strain in neck and shoulders
Contraindications: Lower back, neck, or shoulder injuries

♦ 5. Spread Feet Forward Bend ⊙

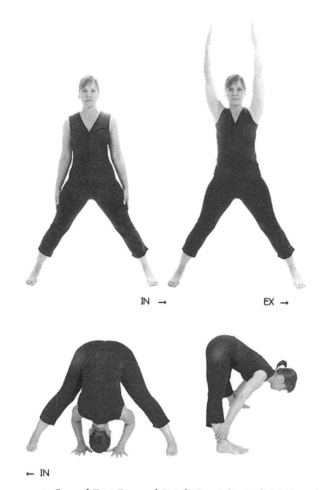

IN →   EX →

← IN

FIGURE 2.5 Spread Feet Forward Bend (*Prasārita Pādottānāsana*)

Sanskrit Name: *Prasārita Pādottānāsana* [prʌ ˈsa rɪ tʌ -
ˈpa dɒt: ta ˈna sʌ nʌ]
Category: Symmetrical Standing Forward Bend
For the Singer: Strengthens legs and back; provides deep stretch
of spinal muscles and inner thigh muscles as well as hamstrings;

works major muscles of the torso, including
the *rectus abdominus* and *obliques* on return to upright
position

Difficulty Level: Beginning

Classic Form: Very wide stance, toes pointing forward, legs
straight, palms down on floor between feet, top of head on floor

***Viniyoga* Adaptations:** Knees may be bent slightly for more
forward rotation of pelvis and deeper stretch of lower back; various
arm positions; top of head toward or on floor

Instructions:

1) Standing in *Samasthiti*, step feet wide apart, bend knees slightly, lift arches
   of feet; exhale completely
2) Inhaling, lift chest to lengthen solar plexus area, raising arms overhead
3) Exhaling, contract abdominal muscles from pubis to navel while bending
   forward with slightly bent knees and weight firmly on heels
4) Keeping upper back as flat as possible and head, arms, and chest aligned
   (or running hands down legs), release into full forward bend
5) Hands may grasp ankles or be placed flat on floor between feet; drop top of
   head toward floor
6) Inhaling, keep abdominals contracted and shift weight to legs, pull chest
   and arms forward and up (or place hands behind back), keeping upper
   back flat, and return to the upright position
7) Exhaling, lower arms to sides

   Common Mistakes: Excessive forward rotation of pelvis;
   collapsing chest over belly; placing weight on balls of feet instead of
   heels; rotation of knees inward or outward; collapsing arches;
   jutting chin

   Risks: Disc compression and muscle strain in lower back; strain in
   neck and shoulders; stress in hip joints

   Contraindications: Lower back problems

♦ **6. Chair Posture** ▶

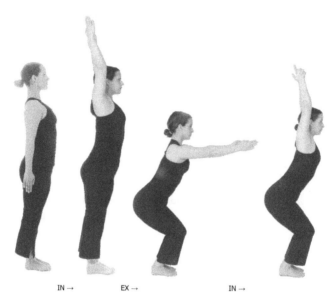

IN →   EX →   IN →

FIGURE 2.6 Chair Posture (*Utkatāsana*)

Sanskrit Name: *Utkatāsana* [ʊt kʌ ˈta sʌ nʌ]
Category: Symmetrical Standing Forward Bend with Knees Bent
For the Singer: Strengthens legs and back for rising from a chair
and standing for long periods; provides strong work in quadriceps,
spinal muscles, and all major abdominal muscles
Difficulty Level: Beginning
Classic Form: A standing forward bend in which the knees are
bent in a half squat, heels remaining on floor, torso upright, arms
overhead with palms together, feet and knees together
***Viniyoga* Adaptations:** Include placing the feet a little apart for
greater stability and deeper squat, and bringing the arms forward
and parallel to the floor or angled upward
Instructions:

1) Stand in *Samasthiti* with feet a little apart, arches lifted; exhale completely
2) Inhaling, raise arms overhead and tuck chin slightly
3) Exhaling, contract the abdominals from pubis to navel and lower buttocks and thighs as though sitting on a chair; keep upper back as erect and flat as possible; arms may remain overhead or in front parallel to floor; keep abdominals tight
4) Inhaling, keeping abdominal muscles contracted, leading with the chest, bring arms and chest forward and up to upright standing position
5) Exhaling, lower arms to sides

> **Common Mistakes:** Common mistakes include lifting heels off floor (though this may be necessary in some cases), collapsing chest over belly, leaning too far forward
> **Risks:** Risks include stress from a tendency to overarch the lower back
> **Contraindications:** Lower back problems, knee problems

♦♦ 7. Intense Side Stretch ▶

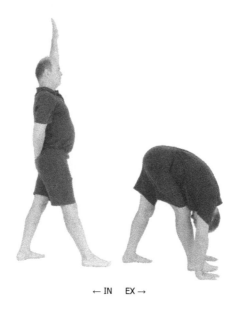

← IN   EX →

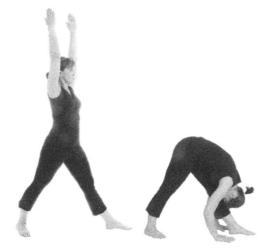

← IN   EX →

FIGURE 2.7 Intense Side Stretch (*Pārśvottānāsana*)

Sanskrit Name: *Pārśvottānāsana* [ˈparʃ voːt ta ˈna sʌ nʌ]
Category: Asymmetrical Standing Forward Bend
For the Singer: Provides deep stretch of hamstrings of one leg
and one side of the back and chest at a time; greatly strengthens
abdominal and back muscles
Difficulty Level: Intermediate
Classic Form: With hands in reverse prayer position (behind the
back), feet stepped wide apart in a walking stance, the torso is
folded forward over the straight front leg until the nose, then lips,
then chin rest below the knee of the front leg
***Viniyoga* Adaptations:** Comfortably wide walking stance; arms
raised overhead on inhale (may fold one arm behind back and raise
only the arm opposite the extended leg to lessen workload on lower
back); front knee slightly bent in forward bend to avoid
overstretching the hamstring, hands on floor on either side of front
foot
Instructions:

1) Standing in *Samasthiti*, take a walking step forward, turning the rear foot
   slightly out for stability; exhale completely
2) Inhaling, raise the arms overhead, lifting the chest; contract the abdominal
   muscles to stabilize the sacrum and protect lower back
3) Exhaling, fold forward over the front leg, front knee slightly bent; place
   hands on floor on either side of the forward foot
4) Inhaling, return to upright position by pulling the chest forward and up,
   arms extended forward or swept up and behind back
5) Exhaling, lower arms to sides
6) Repeat on opposite side

Common Mistakes: Collapsing chest over belly; keeping front
knee locked in the forward bend; lifting chin too high and
compressing cervical spine
Risks: Overstretching lower back and/or hamstring of front leg
Contraindications: Back injury or high blood pressure

◆◆ 8. Half Intense Side Stretch ▶

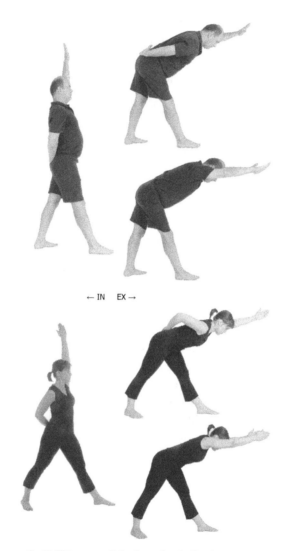

←— IN   EX —→

FIGURE 2.8 Half Intense Side Stretch (*Ardha Pārśvottānāsana*)

Sanskrit Name: *Ardha Pārśvottānāsana* [ˈʌrd hʌ -
ˈparʃ voːt̪ ta ˈna sʌ nʌ]
Category: Asymmetrical Standing Half Forward Bend
For the Singer: Builds strength in the lower abdominal muscles
as they remain contracted throughout the movements of the
posture; primary intention is to build strength in the muscles of the
back and legs
Difficulty Level: Intermediate
Classic Form: Similar to *Ardha Uttānāsana* (4.) except it is
asymmetrical
***Viniyoga* Adaptations:** Slight bending of front knee; use of one
arm at a time
Instructions:

1) Standing in *Samasthiti*, take a walking step forward, turning the rear foot
slightly out for stability, fold arm on side of forward foot behind back and
keep there; exhale completely
2) Inhaling, raise opposite arm overhead
3) Exhaling, contract lower abdominal muscles and fold forward, bringing
chest and belly toward thigh and hand toward opposite foot
4) Inhaling, keeping heels firmly on the floor and leading with the chest, pull
chest and arm forward and up halfway, parallel to the floor; abdominals
remain contracted and upper back flat
5) Exhaling, return to full forward bend
6) Inhaling, keeping abdominals contracted, return to full upright posture
7) Exhaling, lower arm(s)
8) Repeat on opposite side; Variation: May be practiced with both arms
together

Common Mistakes: Excessive forward rotation of pelvis;
collapsing chest over belly; shifting weight to balls of feet; rotation
of knees; collapsing arches; jutting chin forward
Risks: Compression or strain in lower back; strain in neck and
shoulders
Contraindications: Lower back injury

Backward Bends

♦ 9. Warrior (a), (b), (c) ⓑ

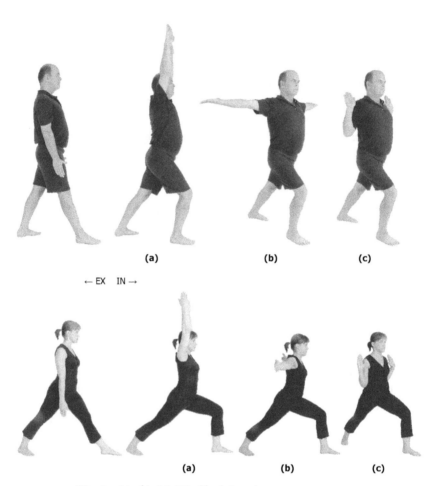

FIGURE 2.9 Warrior (a), (b), (c) (*Vīrabhadrāsana*)

Sanskrit Name: *Vīrabhadrāsana* ['vi rʌb hʌ 'dra sʌ nʌ]
Category: Asymmtrical Standing Backward Bend
For the Singer: Strengthens legs, opens the chest, deepens inhale, strengthens upper and mid-back muscles that keep the chest up
Difficulty Level: Beginning

Classic Form: One foot two shoulders width ahead in a walking stance, front knee bent to align with ankle, back leg straight with heel on floor (foot turned out 45 degrees), chest arched over front thigh, arms straight up with palms together

***Viniyoga* Adaptations:** One foot a comfortable walking step ahead (narrower base); backward bend primarily in the upper back (thoracic spine) rather than in the lower back (lumbar spine); use of arm variations (a, b, c) that open the chest both in repetition and stay

Instructions:

1) Standing in *Samasthiti*, step one foot a big step forward, turning rear foot slightly out for stability; exhale completely
2) Inhaling, press down on the front heel to keep the pelvis back, lift the chest up and forward while raising arms (see variations) and bending the front knee to a position straight over the ankle, being sure the knee tracks straight forward and not to one side; do not push knee beyond the ankle
3) Pulling shoulder blades down and together, arch chest over front thigh, keeping rear heel well grounded, and tuck chin slightly
4) Exhaling, contract abdominal muscles and bring arms partly or fully downward while straightening the knee
5) Repeat on opposite side

Arm variations: a) Arms straight overhead, palms facing forward or toward each other; b) arms forward, up, then out horizontally, palms up; c) elbows bent and arms pulled back so that forward-facing palms are in line with or behind shoulders. Each successive variation increases the work of the shoulder blade muscles.

Common Mistakes: Overarching the lower back (lumbar spine); lifting rear heel; shifting weight to front leg; collapsing or overextending the neck

Risks: Compression of lower back; strain in neck and shoulder muscles; stress in the front knee by bending beyond the ankle; possible stress in hip joints

Contraindications: High blood pressure, heart problems; shoulder or neck problems can be accommodated with arm and head adaptations

Lateral Bends

♦ **10. Extended Triangle** ▶

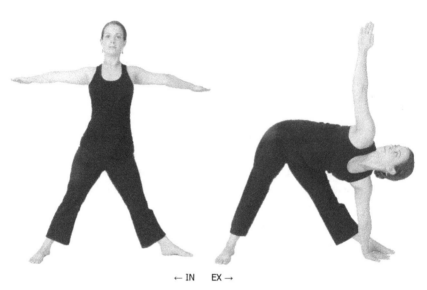

← IN   EX →

FIGURE 2.10 Extended Triangle (*Utthita Trikoṇāsana*)

Sanskrit Name: *Utthita Trikoṇāsana* [ʊtːt ˈhɪ tʌ -
trɪ ko ˈna sʌ nʌ]
Category: Asymmetrical Standing Lateral Bend with Straight
Knee
For the Singer: Deep stretching of the sides of the body, including
intercostals and connective tissue of rib cage; opens hips for greater
flexibility; provides strong stretch of shoulder girdle and deep spinal
muscles
Difficulty Level: Beginning
Classic Form: A wide stance, one foot turned 90 degrees outward,
lateral bend in the direction of the turned foot, hand on that side flat
on floor behind foot, opposite arm raised straight up, fingers
pointing upward, head turned toward the upward hand

***Viniyoga* Adaptations:** Slight bending of the knee on the outward turned leg, turning head down; lower hand above or below knee, palm out; use of arm variations

Instructions:

1) Standing in *Samasthiti* sideways on the mat, step feet apart in a wide stance and turn one foot 90 degrees outward, keeping the pelvis squared forward; exhale completely
2) Inhaling, raise the arm of the turned side overhead, then the other arm horizontally, rotated outward and slightly back or both arms horizontally
3) Exhaling, contract abdominal and gluteus muscles, and bend torso sideways toward the turned foot, bending the knee slightly, keeping arms in a straight line
4) Keep pelvis in place, not displaced forward, backward, or toward the bend, and shoulders facing forward; place hand at or below knee, palm out
5) Inhaling, lift lower arm and return to upright position
6) Exhaling, lower arms to sides
7) Repeat on opposite side

Common Mistakes: Collapsing chest over belly; displacement of pelvis; rotating top shoulder forward; inward rotation of ankles and knees; collapsing arches of feet

Risks: Stress in the lower back, hip joints, neck, and shoulders

Contraindications: Low blood pressure; shoulder or hip injury

♦♦ 11. Extended Lateral Angle or Standing Side Angle ▶

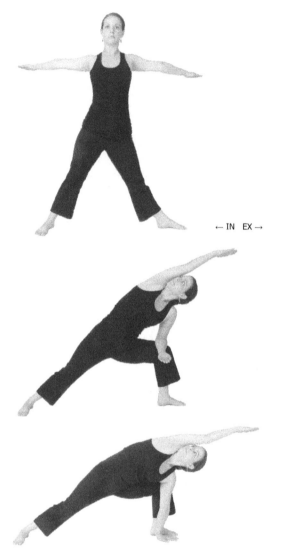

← IN   EX →

FIGURE 2.11 Extended Lateral Angle (*Utthita Pārśva Koṇāsana*)

Sanskrit Name: *Utthita Pārśva Koṇāsana* [ʊtːt ˈhɪ tʌ - ˈparʃ vʌ - ko ˈna sʌ nʌ]

Category: Asymmetrical Standing Lateral Bend with Bent Knee

For the Singer: Strong stretch of the sides of the body, including lower ribs; opens hips for greater flexibility; contributes to leg strength

Difficulty Level: Intermediate

Classic Form: Very wide stance, one foot turned outward 90 degrees; knee is brought over ankle of turned foot, thigh parallel to the floor, hand flat on floor outside turned foot, opposite arm pulled straight over ear, head turned to look up at the hand; body is in a single plane

***Viniyoga* Adaptations:** Approach the posture with repetitions of the lateral bend before staying in the posture; rest elbow on thigh of leg with turned foot; bring upper arm somewhat behind torso to help rotate chest upward; arm adaptations coordinated with breath (inhale arm straight over ear; exhale arm back to side of body)

Instructions:

1) Standing in *Samasthiti* sideways on the mat, step feet apart in a wide stance and turn one foot 90 degrees outward; exhale completely
2) Inhaling, raise arms to horizontal; contract the abdominals
3) Exhaling, bend the outward turned knee to a position straight over the ankle and the torso laterally, keeping hips in place, until the elbow can rest on the thigh parallel to the floor; keep back leg straight and outside of foot pressed onto the floor
4) Inhaling, bring the top arm straight over the ear, rotating the chest toward the ceiling until the whole body is in a single plane from heel to fingertips; look up at hand or down at foot
5) Exhaling, stabilize the posture
6) Inhaling, straighten the knee and return the arms to horizontal
7) Exhaling, lower arms to sides
8) Repeat on opposite side

Common Mistakes: Bent knee goes beyond the ankle or falls inward or outward and does not track straight forward; chest collapses forward over belly; head comes forward and chest rolls toward floor; foot of straight leg rolls inward; abdominal muscles remain slack

Risks: Stress on bent knee; torque of lower back if chest rolls forward; loss of balance

Contraindications: High or low blood pressure; knee, hip, or shoulder injury

Twists

♦ 12. Revolved Triangle ⓘ

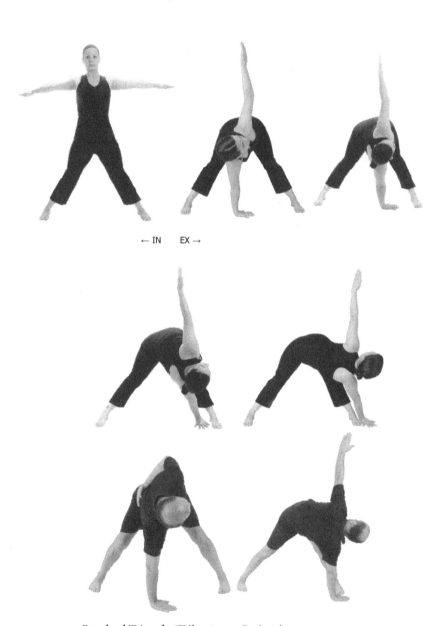

← IN   EX →

FIGURE 2.12 Revolved Triangle (*Trikoṇāsana Parivṛtti*)

Sanskrit Name: *Trikoṇāsana Parivṛtti* [ˈtrɪ ko ˈna sʌ nʌ - pʌ rɪ ˈvrtː tɪ]

Category: Asymmetrical Standing Twist

For the Singer: Enhances spinal flexibility; works muscles of shoulder girdle, relieving tightness in the shoulders; strengthens muscles of the pelvic girdle and legs

Difficulty Level: Beginning

Classic Form: Feet wide apart, toes pointing forward (or one foot turned 90 degrees outward); torso twisted forward with arms and shoulders aligned vertically (shoulders stacked), downward hand flat on floor outside opposite foot, fingers pointing forward; head turned up to look at upper hand

Viniyoga Adaptations: Feet remain forward; gradual moving of hand on floor from the center position to the outside of the opposite foot with four repetitions; may fold upper arm behind back for a deeper rotation of the shoulder girdle; slight bending of opposite knee for more twisting rotation

Instructions:

1) Standing in *Samasthiti* sideways on the mat, step feet wide apart, toes facing forward; exhale completely
2) Inhaling, lift chest and raise arms to horizontal position
3) Exhaling, tighten lowest abdominal muscles, pulling pubic bone upward, and begin twisting while bending forward; press outsides of feet into the floor
4) Place hand flat on floor in the center between the feet, fingers pointing toward opposite foot
5) Align (stack) the shoulder girdle and upward pointing arm in a straight line over the hand on the floor; face upward
6) Inhaling, lift arms and return to upright position
7) Repeat three more times, moving hand on floor closer to opposite foot and finally outside the foot, fingers pointing forward or to the side
8) After last repetition, exhale and lower arms
9) Repeat to other side

Common Mistakes: Hip displacement forward or to the side; inward rotation of leg or pivoting of heel opposite the twist (for some body structures, this displacement may be necessary to protect the lower back); moving hand but not shoulders toward opposite foot; collapsing arches of the feet

Risks: Shear stress in knees or sacrum; muscle strain in neck and shoulders; compression of spine

Contraindications: Back or spine injury; low blood pressure; migraine; dizziness or vertigo

Balance

♦♦ 13. Mountain (with balance variations a. and b.) ⊙

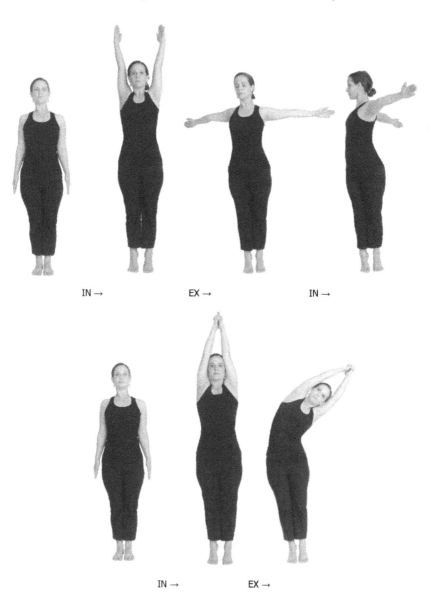

IN →   EX →   IN →

IN →   EX →

FIGURE 2.13 Mountain with Balance Variations (*Tāḍāsana*)

Sanskrit Name: *Tāḍāsana* [ta ˈda sʌ nʌ]

Category: Asymmetrical Standing Balance Postures

For the Singer: All standing balance postures promote a focused and stable mind and, secondarily, contribute to leg and torso strength as well as to good balance in any position; develops physical and mental confidence

Difficulty Level: Intermediate

Viniyoga* Adaptation:** This series is an adaptation of ***Tāḍāsana as two-footed or toe balances

Instructions:

1) Stand in *Samasthiti* and exhale completely
2) Inhaling, raise arms overhead and heels high off floor so that the balance is on the toes
3) Exhaling, extend arms out horizontally, remaining on toes
4) Inhaling, turn body to one side and head to the other or same side
5) Exhaling, return to center; inhaling, repeat to opposite side (a)
6) Inhaling, raise arms overhead to form a circle at fingertips and bend to one side, still balancing on toes and looking up (b)
7) Exhaling, return to center; inhaling, repeat to opposite side
8) Exhaling, lower arms to sides and heels to floor

Common Mistakes: Not coming all the way up onto toes

Risks: Loss of balance

Contraindications: Weak ankles and feet; dizziness or vertigo

◆◆ **14. Tree** ▶

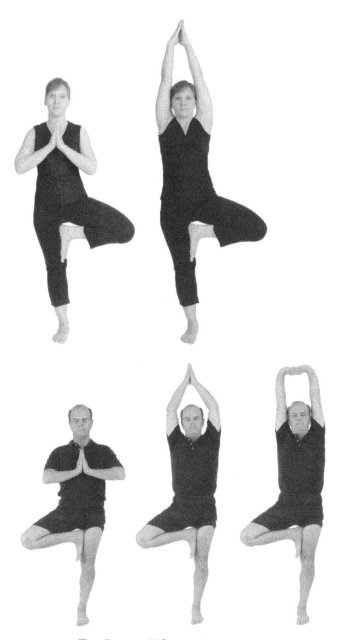

FIGURE 2.14 Tree Posture (*Vṛkṣāsana*)

Sanskrit Name: *Vṛkṣāsana* [vr ˈkʃa sʌ nʌ]
Category: Asymmetrical Standing Balance Posture
For the Singer: Develops a focused and stable mind; contributes to leg and torso strength; develops physical and mental confidence
Difficulty Level: Intermediate
Classic Form: One leg is bent, sole of foot flat against upper thigh of opposite leg, knee turned out at a right angle, arms straight overhead with palms together, entire balance on standing leg
***Viniyoga* Adaptations:** Palms together at chest
Instructions:

1) Stand in *Samasthiti;* focus eyes at a point in front and slightly down; shift weight to the side of leg balance; tighten lower abdominal and gluteus muscles
2) Place the sole of opposite foot firmly against the thigh of the balancing leg above the knee, at the groin if possible, using hands for placement if necessary
3) Inhaling, bring hands together at chest or raise above head, palms together
4) Stay in posture for several breaths
5) Exhaling, lower arms to sides and foot to floor
6) Repeat on the opposite side

> **Common Mistakes:** Forgetting to contract lowest abdominal muscles before entering posture; hip displacement to side or back; collapsing chest over belly; jutting chin forward; inward or outward rotation of supporting leg
> **Risks:** Compression or strain in lower back; stress in hip, knee, or ankle joints
> **Contraindications:** Low or high blood pressure; dizziness or vertigo

♦♦♦ 15. One-Footed Standing Big Toe Holding Posture

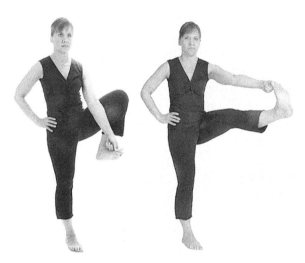

FIGURE 2.15 One-Footed Standing Big Toe Holding Posture (*Utthita Eka Pādāṅguṣṭhāsana*)

Sanskrit Name: *Utthita Eka Pādāṅguṣṭhāsana* [ʊtːt ˈhɪ tʌ - ˈe kʌ - ˈpa daŋ gʊʃt ˈha sʌ nʌ]
Category: Asymmetrical Standing Balance Posture
For the Singer: Develops a focused and stable mind; contributes to leg and torso strength; develops physical and mental confidence
Difficulty Level: Intermediate/Advanced
Classic Form: Standing on one leg, same side hand on the hip, the opposite leg is stretched straight forward, hand grasping the toes of the outstretched leg; spine is erect; chin is level
***Viniyoga* Adaptations:** None
Instructions:

1) Stand in *Samasthiti;* focus eyes at a point in front and slightly down; shift weight to the side of leg balance, tighten abdominal muscles, and place same side hand on hip; exhale completely
2) Inhaling, lift chest and extend spine
3) Exhaling, bend knee and lift leg until thigh is parallel to floor
4) Inhaling, grasp big toe with other hand and straighten leg out in front
5) Stay in position for several breaths
6) Inhaling, release toe and lower leg to floor
7) Repeat on opposite side

Common Mistakes: See 14.

Risks: Compression or strain in lower back; stress in hip, knee, or ankle joints

Contraindications: Lower back or ankle injuries; dizziness or vertigo

♦♦ **16. Warrior, Balance Variation** ▶

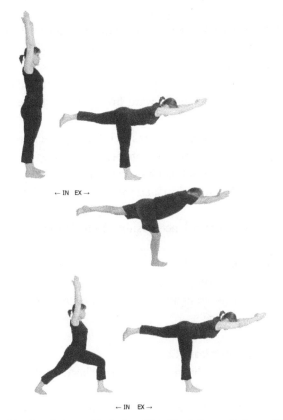

FIGURE 2.16 Warrior, Balance Variation (*Vīrabhadrāsana*, Balance Variation)

Sanskrit Name: *Vīrabhadrāsana,* Balance Variation
['vi rʌb hʌ 'dra sʌ nʌ]
Category: Asymmetrical Standing Balance Posture
For the Singer: Develops a focused and stable mind; greatly
strengthens leg and torso muscles; develops physical and mental
confidence
Difficulty Level: Intermediate
Classic Form: Entire body is balanced on one leg, the opposite leg,
torso, and extended arms, palms together, aligned parallel to the
floor; head is lifted to face forward
***Viniyoga* Adaptations:** Head remains aligned with spine, facing
downward
Instructions:

1) Standing in *Samasthiti,* step forward into Warrior stance, arms at sides;
   exhale completely
2) Inhaling, raise arms overhead, palms facing, and bend front knee to a right
   angle over the ankle; tighten lower abdominal muscles
3) Exhaling, lift back leg and fold torso forward while straightening the bent
   knee, arms straight forward in alignment with torso and leg, head facing
   downward
4) Or, exhale directly into balance posture from *Samasthiti* with arms overhead
5) Stay in posture for several breaths
6) Inhaling, return to upright stance
7) Exhaling, lower arms, straighten front leg, and step back
8) Repeat on opposite side

Common Mistakes: See 14.
Risks: Compression or strain in lower back; stress in hip, knee, or
ankle joints
Contraindications: High blood pressure; dizziness or vertigo

♦♦♦ 17. One-Footed Forward Bend ▶

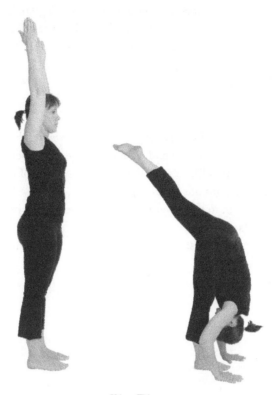

← IN   EX →

FIGURE 2.17 One-Footed Forward Bend (*Ekapāda Uttānāsana*)

Sanskrit Name: *Ekapāda Uttānāsana* [e kʌ ˈpa dʌ - ʊtː ta ˈna sʌ nʌ]

For the Singer: Develops strength in the leg, back, and gluteus muscles; contributes to good balance in a forward bend

Difficulty Level: Advanced

Classic Form: Both legs straight; opposite hand grasps ankle of standing leg; other hand flat on floor; lifted leg straight up with toes pointed upward; head on knee of standing leg

***Viniyoga* Adaptations:** Both hands on floor on either side of foot; lifted leg at an obtuse angle with the floor rather than vertical

Instructions:

1) Standing in *Samasthiti*, inhale and raise arms overhead; tighten lower abdominal muscles
2) Exhaling, come into a forward bend, raising one leg straight out behind and as far up to vertical as possible, both hands on the floor to either side of the foot, head to knee or shin; stay several breaths
3) Inhaling, return to upright position
4) Exhaling, lower arms to sides
5) Repeat on opposite side

Common Mistakes: Failing to contract lowest abdominal muscles to initiate the forward bend; collapsing chest over belly; displacement of hips to the side or back; twisting of torso; inward or outward rotation of supporting leg
Risks: Strain in the lower back; shear stress in the hip, knee, ankle, or sacroiliac joints
Contraindications: Lower back problems; low or high blood pressure

Kneeling

Axial Extension

♦ 18. Downward Facing Dog ▶

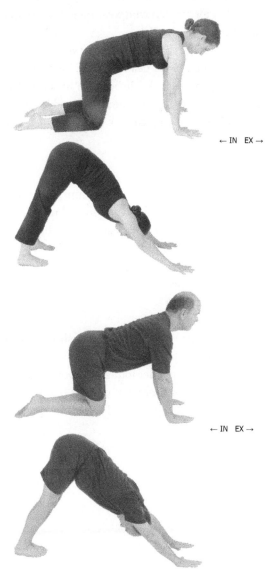

← IN   EX →

← IN   EX →

FIGURE 2.18 Downward Facing Dog (*Adho Mukha Śvānāsana*)

Sanskrit Name: *Adho Mukha Śvānāsana* [ˈʌd ho ˈmʊk hʌ - ʃva ˈna sʌ nʌ]

Category: Symmetrical Axial Extension Posture

For the Singer: Excellent for extending spine, flattening upper back, strengthening shoulders, stretching legs, especially calves and achilles tendon for women who wear high heels frequently

Difficulty Level: Beginning

Classic Form: Hands and feet at a very wide angle, knees tight, feet flat on the floor, top of head on floor; intense stretch

***Viniyoga* Adaptations:** Angle between hands and feet less wide, hips pushed back over legs as much as possible, heels as close to floor as possible, head aligned with spine between arms, knees slightly bent

Instructions:

1) Beginning on hands and knees, knees under hips, hands under shoulders, toes turned under, inhale and contract abdominal muscles
2) Exhaling, press down on arms and feet and lift hips straight up; turn creases of elbows forward to engage shoulder blade muscles
3) Bring chest toward feet, hips over legs, heels to floor (or as close as possible), ears between elbows; do not hyperextend shoulders
4) Inhaling, return knees to floor

Common Mistakes: Hyperextension of shoulders; excessive forward rotation of pelvis causing compression in the lower back

Risks: Stress in the shoulder joints; compression in lower back if alignment not straight; stress to the wrists or elbows

Contraindications: Carpal tunnel syndrome, pregnancy, high blood pressure, or headache

Forward Bends

♦ **19. Ruddy Goose with Child's Pose** ▶

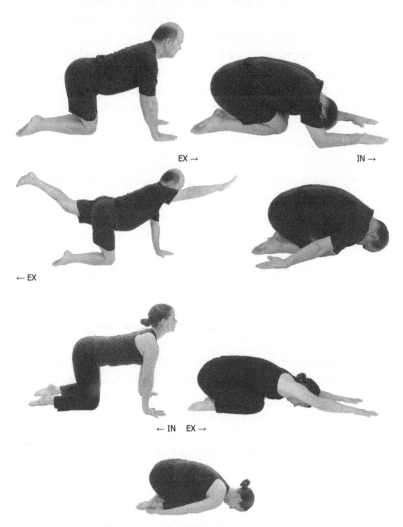

EX →   IN →

← EX

← IN   EX →

FIGURE 2.19 Ruddy Goose with Child's Pose (*Cakravākāsana*)

Sanskrit Name: *Cakravākāsana* ['tʃʌ krʌ va 'ka sʌ nʌ]
Category: Symmetrical Kneeling Forward Bend
For the Singer: A safe and effective stretch of the lower back and neck; useful for lengthening and controlling exhalation
Difficulty Level: Beginning
Classic Form: An adaptation of a classic backward bend
***Viniyoga* Adaptation:** Hands and knees on floor, feet pointing straight backward, hands under the shoulders, knees slightly apart under hips, torso parallel to floor, elbows slightly bent, back slightly concave, head raised
Instructions:

1) Kneeling with hands on floor, palms down under shoulders, knees slightly apart under hips, exhale completely
2) Inhaling, lift chest and head and slightly sink the lower back
3) Exhaling, tuck chin, contract lowest abdominal muscles, rounding the lower back, and begin lowering buttocks to heels, bending elbows to floor first, then chest to thighs and head to floor; hands remain on floor (knees may be wider apart if needed)
4) Inhaling, pressing down palms, pull chest forward and up, shoulders slightly down and back, straightening elbows near the end of the movement
5) Staying in position, contract abdominals, lift chest and chin slightly higher
   Arm and Leg Adaptations: inhale forward to hands and knees and lift one leg and the opposite arm straight out; exhale, bringing arm and leg back to position and continue into Child's Pose

Common Mistakes: Bending only from hips; keeping elbows straight; collapsing chest over belly; rolling heels out; jutting chin forward
Risks: Cumulative stress in wrists and knees; compression in lower back or neck; muscle strain in neck
Contraindications: Knee injury; diarrhea; pregnancy

♦ **20. Kneeling Forward Bend** ▶

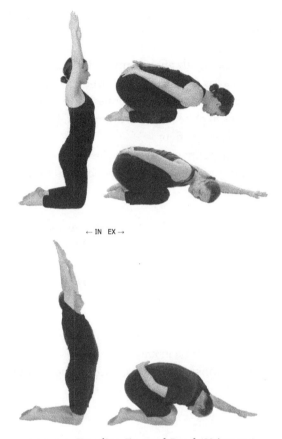

← IN EX →

FIGURE 2.20 Kneeling Forward Bend (*Vajrāsana*)

Sanskrit Name: *Vajrāsana* [vʌdʒ 'ra sʌ nʌ]
Category: Symmetrical Kneeling Forward Bend
For the Singer: A safe stretch for the spinal muscles; strong work
in the spinal muscles and quadriceps coming out of the posture;
increases flexibility in muscles of the shoulder girdle; strengthens
connection between lower and upper spine; expands chest with arm
variation
Difficulty Level: Beginning
Classic Form: An adaptation of a seated meditation posture

Viniyoga **Adaptation:** Sit bones on heels, knees slightly apart, torso flat on thighs, hands palms up on lower back, forehead on floor

Instructions:

1) Stand erect on knees slightly apart, arms at sides; exhale completely
2) Inhaling, lift chest away from belly, raise arms overhead, tuck chin
3) Exhaling, contract lowest abdominal muscles to initiate forward bend, sweeping arms back to place hands on lower back, lower buttocks to heels, chest to thighs, forehead to floor
4) Inhaling, abdominals contracted, sweep arms out and up while lifting chest to upright kneeling position, keeping upper back as flat as possible
5) Exhaling, lower arms

Variation: While bending forward, extend one arm forward and sweep the other to the back, turning head in the direction of the back arm; repeat, alternating arms and head turns

Common Mistakes: Collapsing chest over belly; rounding upper back; jutting chin, rolling heels outward; allowing knees to come apart

Risks: Stress in lower back, neck, or shoulders; compression in neck; cumulative stress in knees

Contraindications: Lower back, neck, or shoulder problems; knee injury

♦♦♦ 21. One-Footed Pigeon King (with Forward Bend Variation) ⊙

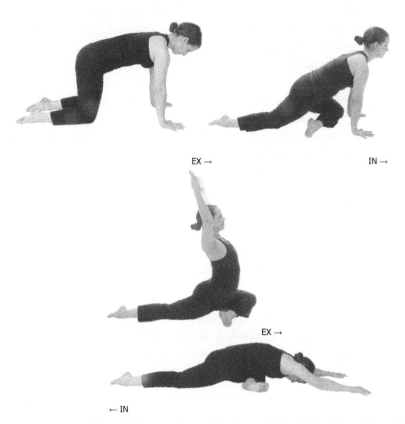

FIGURE 2.21 One-Footed Pigeon King with Forward Bend Variation (*Ekapāda Rājakapotāsana*)

Sanskrit Name: *Ekapāda Rājakapotāsana* [e kʌ ˈpa dʌ - ˈra dʒʌ kʌ po ˈta sʌ nʌ]

Category: Asymmetrical Kneeling Backward Bend with Forward Bend Variation

For the Singer: Strongly stretches hip rotator muscles in the bent leg; stretches psoas muscle in the straight leg; works upper back muscles that keep the chest up and open

Difficulty Level: Advanced

Classic Form: One leg bent, heel at groin, knee on floor; other leg extended straight out behind, top of shin, knee, and foot on floor;

chest pushed out as far as possible, hands on floor; then bend straight leg, bringing lower leg perpendicular to the floor, grasp ankle with one hand, then both, and bring close to head

Viniyoga Adaptations: Less extreme chest position; hands remain on floor, helping to arch the upper back; exhalation phase becomes a forward bend over the bent leg

Instructions:

1) Beginning on hands and knees, bring left knee up to left hand and left foot close to right hand
2) Extend right leg straight back with left hip on the floor; hands are on floor on either side of bent leg; exhale completely
3) Inhaling, lift rib cage forward and up, pulling down and back with hands to push chest forward, flattening upper back
4) Exhaling, lower chest to bent leg and forehead to floor
5) Inhaling return to upright position
6) Exhaling, return to hands and knees
7) Repeat on opposite side

Common Mistakes: Excessive arching of lumbar spine; collapsing neck backward; shrugging shoulders up toward ears; rounding forward or hyperextending shoulder joints

Risks: Strain in neck and lower back; excessive disc compression

Contraindications: Lower back, ankle, or knee injury; tight hips or thighs

Backward Bends

♦ ♦ 22. Lizard (with Forward Bend Variation) ▶

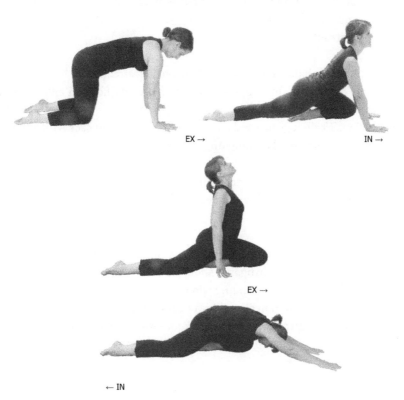

FIGURE 2.22 Lizard (*Godhāpīṭham*)

Sanskrit Name: *Godhāpīṭham* [god ha ˈpit hʌm]
Category: Asymmetrical Kneeling Backward Bend with Forward
Bend Variation
For the Singer: Stretches front of torso, especially the psoas
muscle, and opens the chest; flattens the thoracic curve and works
the upper back muscles responsible for keeping chest up and open
during singing
Difficulty Level: Intermediate
Classic Form: One leg folded underneath, the other leg stretched
straight out behind, top of foot on floor, arms straight, hands on

either side of folded leg, chest pushed as forward as possible, head back

***Viniyoga* Adaptations:** In repetition, on exhale lower chest to thigh and head to floor; chest position less extreme; head level with chin slightly tucked

Instructions:

1) Beginning on hands and knees, extend one leg straight out behind, bending the other knee until hips are on foot; hands on floor on either side of bent knee; exhale completely
2) Inhaling, lift rib cage forward and up, pulling down and back with hands to push chest forward, flattening upper back
3) Exhaling, lower chest to thigh, forehead to floor
4) Inhaling, return to upright position
5) Exhaling, return to hands and knees
6) Repeat on opposite side

Common Mistakes: Excessive arching of lumbar spine; collapsing neck backward; shrugging shoulders up toward ears; rounding forward or hyperextending shoulder joints

Risks: Strain in neck and lower back; excessive disc compression

Contraindications: Knee, neck, or lower back injury

♦♦♦ **23. Camel** ⊚

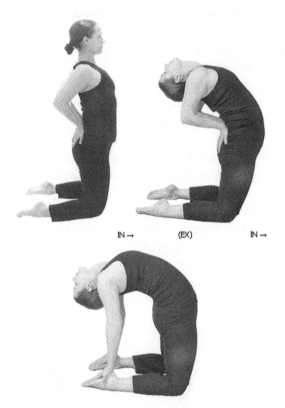

IN →   (EX)   IN →

FIGURE 2.23 Camel (*Uṣṭrāsana*)

Sanskrit Name: *Uṣṭrāsana* [ʊʃ ˈtra sʌ nʌ]
Category: Symmetrical Kneeling Backward Bend—Fixed Frame
For the Singer: Strong stretch for the front of the body; expands the chest, flattens the upper back, and deepens the arch of the lower back
Difficulty Level: Advanced
Classic Form: Knees and feet together, thighs perpendicular to the floor, spine arched backward with hands on soles of feet, chest parallel to the ceiling, neck extended
***Viniyoga* Adaptations:** Knees may be slightly apart; toes may be tucked under for a less deep arch of the back

Instructions:

1) Kneel on the floor, torso upright, hands on back of pelvis; exhale completely
2) Inhaling, lift chest away from belly, pulling shoulder blades together and arching upper back; exhale; inhaling, reach back with one hand at a time and grasp heels, or place hands on soles of feet (if arms are too short to reach feet, turn toes under to raise heels)
3) Stay in posture for a few breaths, refining the arch of the upper back
4) Exhaling, release hands one at a time and return torso to upright

> **Common Mistakes:** Leading with the head; failing to contract shoulder blade muscles; hyperflexing the shoulder muscles
> **Risks:** Strain to the lower back and neck; strain in the shoulders from hyperextension
> **Contraindications:** Lower back, neck, or shoulder injury; high or low blood pressure; migraine

♦♦♦ **24. One-Footed Camel** ▶

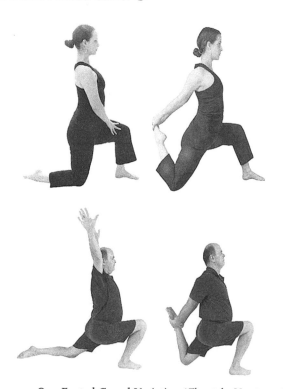

FIGURE 2.24 One-Footed Camel Variation (*Ekapāda Uṣṭrāsana*)

Sanskrit Name: *Ekapāda Uṣṭrāsana* [e kʌ ˈpa dʌ - ʊʃ ˈtra sʌ nʌ]
Category: Asymmetrical Kneeling Backward Bend—Fixed Frame
For the Singer: Strong stretch of the psoas and upper thigh
muscles; opens the chest; works muscles of upper back and
shoulders
Difficulty Level: Advanced
Classic Form: One knee on floor, leg straight back, top of foot on
floor; other leg bent at the knee, foot flat on floor; spine arched
backward with arms straight, one hand on sole of foot, other hand
on floor beside foot; neck extended
***Viniyoga* Adaptations:** Front knee in a deeper bend, torso
upright, extended leg bent with both hands grasping the sole of the
foot, arms straight, head upright, chin slightly tucked
Instructions:

1) Kneeling, bring one foot forward flat on the floor slightly ahead of the knee;
   place both hands on bent knee; opposite leg is stretched straight out behind,
   top of foot on floor; exhale completely
2) Inhaling, lift chest away from belly, bend extended leg to bring foot to a
   vertical position; reach back one hand at a time and grasp the top of the
   foot, arms straight
3) Stay in posture for a few breaths
4) Exhaling, release hands one at a time, lower foot to floor, and return to
   kneeling position
5) Repeat on opposite side

Common Mistakes: Overarching the lower back; collapsing neck
backward; hyperextending shoulders
Risks: Strain to the lower back, neck, and shoulders
Contraindications: Lower back, neck, shoulder, or knee injury

Prone

Backward Bends

♦ **25. Cobra** ⊙

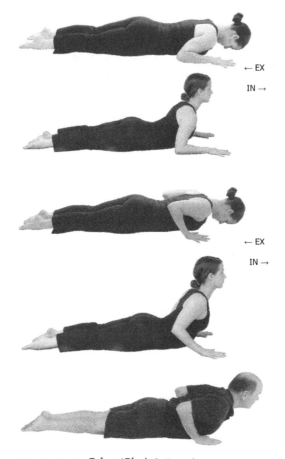

FIGURE 2.25 Cobra (*Bhujaṅgāsana*)

Sanskrit Name: *Bhujaṅgāsana* [bhʊ dʒʌŋ ˈga sʌ nʌ]
Category: Symmetrical Prone Backward Bend
For the Singer: Greatly strengthens the muscles of the upper back
that keep the chest up throughout a sung phrase; also strengthens
the lower abdominal muscles, which remain contracted throughout
the posture
Difficulty Level: Beginning
Classic Form: Legs together; palms on floor at waist, elbows up;
chest lifted to point of pubis; head faces forward

***Viniyoga* Adaptations:** Legs slightly apart to protect lower back; hands slightly ahead of shoulders, forearms on floor, to assist the opening of the chest; chest lifted only to point of navel to increase work in the upper back muscles and protect lower back

Instructions:

1) Lying on stomach, legs slightly apart, palms down slightly in front of shoulders, forearms on floor; forehead on floor, exhale completely, contracting abdominal muscles
2) Inhaling, pull back on hands and forearms to pull shoulder blade muscles together and down, lifting chest forward and up (do not push up with arms)
3) Keeping legs on floor and shoulder blades down and together, push sternum forward and lift head to face forward
4) Exhaling, look down, contract abdominals, and lower chest and forehead to floor

> **Common Mistakes:** Pushing chest up with arm leverage; excessive arch in lower back; lifting legs; leading with the head; raising shoulders; lifting elbows off floor
>
> **Risks:** Compression or muscle strain in the lower back; compression or muscle strain in the neck
>
> **Contraindications:** Lower back injury; pregnancy

♦ **26. Locust** ▶

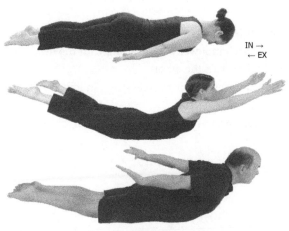

IN →
← EX

FIGURE 2.26 Locust (*Śalabhāsana*)

Sanskrit Name: *Śalabhāsana* [ʃʌ lʌb 'ha sʌ nʌ]
Category: Symmetrical Prone Backbend
For the Singer: Greatly strengthens the spinal and gluteus muscles; opens the chest; stretches the whole front of the body; strengthens abdominal muscles that remain contracted throughout the movements in the posture
Difficulty Level: Beginning
Classic Form: Chest and legs lifted off floor; arms lifted straight forward, palms together; head lifted to face forward
***Viniyoga* Adaptations:** Legs slightly apart; beginning arm position places hands palms up on the sacrum; head turned to one side; legs should not be lifted higher than chest; arms lifted back
Instructions:

1) Lying on stomach, legs together or slightly apart, place hands palms up on sacrum and turn head to one side, resting cheek on floor; exhale completely; contract lower abdominals and pull shoulder blades together and down the back
2) Inhaling, pull chest forward and up, lift both legs only to chest height, lifting arms or sweeping arms forward or out to the sides and turning head to center
3) Lengthen back of neck, push sternum forward, and lift head to face forward
4) Exhaling, lower chest and legs to floor, returning arms to original position and turning head to the opposite side, resting cheek on floor

Common Mistakes: Legs open too wide or lifted too high causing excessive arch in lower back; leading with the head; lifting one arm or leg higher than the other
Risks: Compression or muscle strain in lower back or neck; stress in shoulders
Contraindications: Lower back, shoulder, or neck injury; pregnancy

♦ 27. Half Locust ⊙

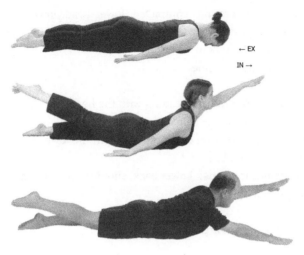

← EX

IN →

FIGURE 2.27 Half Locust (*Ardha Śalabhāsana*)

Sanskrit Name: *Ardha Śalabhāsana* [ˈʌrd hʌ - ʃʌ lʌb ˈha sʌ nʌ]
Category: Asymmetrical Prone Backbend
For the Singer: Strengthens the spinal, gluteus, and shoulder
girdle muscles one side at a time; works opposite sides of body and
both sides of the brain at the same time; strengthens abdominal
muscles as they remain contracted throughout the movements of
the posture
Difficulty Level: Beginning
Classic Form: Upper torso, one leg, and the opposite arm are lifted
off the floor; arm is straight out in front while other arm rests on
floor at the side; head is lifted forward
***Viniyoga* Adaptations:** Legs slightly apart; arms may be placed
palms up on sacrum; leg is lifted no higher than chest
Instructions:

1) Lying on stomach with legs together or slightly apart, rest arms at sides or
   palms up on the sacrum; turn head to one side; exhale completely; tighten
   abdominal muscles and pull shoulder blades together and down the back
2) Inhaling, pull chest forward and up, sweeping one arm forward, turning
   head to center, and lifting the opposite leg no higher than the chest

3) Extend head away from shoulders without lifting chin; gently push sternum forward, then lift head to face forward

4) Exhaling, with abdominals contracted, lower head, lower chest, leg, and arm to original position on floor, turning the head in the opposite direction, resting cheek on floor

5) Repeat on the opposite side

> **Common Mistakes:** Leading with the head; lifting leg higher than chest; rolling to one side
>
> **Risks:** Compression or muscle strain in the lower back or neck; stress in shoulders
>
> **Contraindications:** Lower back, shoulder, or neck injury; pregnancy

♦ 28. Chariot or Airplane Posture ▶

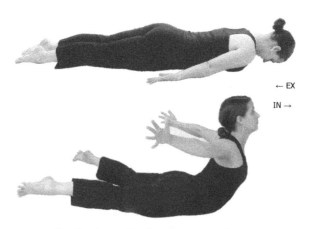

← EX

IN →

FIGURE 2.28 Chariot or Airplane Posture (*Vimānāsana*)

> **Sanskrit Name:** *Vimānāsana* [vɪ ma ˈna sʌ nʌ]
>
> **Category:** Symmetrical Prone Backward Bend
>
> **For the Singer:** Strengthens all the musculature that supports the lower back as well as strongly working the outer thigh muscles, gluteus, spinal, and hip rotator muscles; abdominal muscles are also strongly worked by remaining contracted throughout
>
> **Difficulty Level:** Beginning

Classic Form: Upper torso, arms, and legs are lifted off the floor, the arms and legs spread wide, head lifted to face forward
Viniyoga **Adaptations:** Legs should be lifted no higher than the chest; arm spread should be equal to or greater than the spread of the legs
Instructions:

1) Lying on stomach with legs together or slightly apart, rest arms at sides or palms up on the sacrum; turn head to one side; exhale completely; tighten abdominal muscles and pull shoulder blades together and down the back
2) Inhaling, pull chest forward and up, sweeping arms wide and lifting and spreading the legs wide, no higher than the chest
3) Extend head away from shoulders without lifting chin; gently push sternum forward, and then lift head to face forward
4) Exhaling, with abdominals contracted, lower chest, legs, and arms to original position on floor, turning the head in the opposite direction, resting cheek on floor

> **Common Mistakes:** Leading with the head; legs lifted higher than chest, creating too much arch in the lower back; lifting one leg higher than the other
> **Risks:** Compression or muscle strain in lower back or neck and shoulders; stress in sacroiliac or hip joints
> **Contraindications:** Lower back, shoulder, or neck injury; pregnancy

♦♦ **29. Bow** ⓹

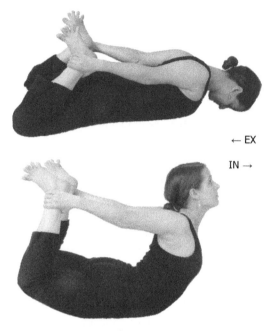

← EX

IN →

FIGURE 2.29 Bow (*Dhanurāsana*)

Sanskrit Name: *Dhanurāsana* [dhʌ nʊ ˈra sʌ nʌ]
Category: Prone Symmetrical Backward Bend—Fixed Frame
For the Singer: Strongly expands chest, stretches front of torso, flattens upper back, stretches shoulders and quadriceps; stay position greatly strengthens abdominal muscles
Difficulty Level: Intermediate
Classic Form: Entire body rests only on the abdomen—ribs and pelvis do not touch floor; arms are straight as hands grasp ankles; after coming into position, knees and ankles are brought together; head is back as far as possible
***Viniyoga* Adaptations:** Arch of back less deep; head kept in line with spine; pelvis may remain on floor
Instructions:

1) Lying face down, bend knees and bring feet close to buttocks, grasp ankles with hands; exhaling completely, contract lower abdominal muscles
2) Inhaling, press feet back, pull shoulders back, and lift chest and knees off floor simultaneously
3) Exhaling, return to beginning position

Common Mistakes: Collapsing spine toward floor; dropping head forward; putting too much pressure on heels of hands; hyperextending shoulders

Risks: Stress to wrists, shoulders, lower back, neck

Contraindications: Lower back, shoulder, or wrist injury; pregnancy

♦ ♦ 30. Upward Facing Dog ⊙

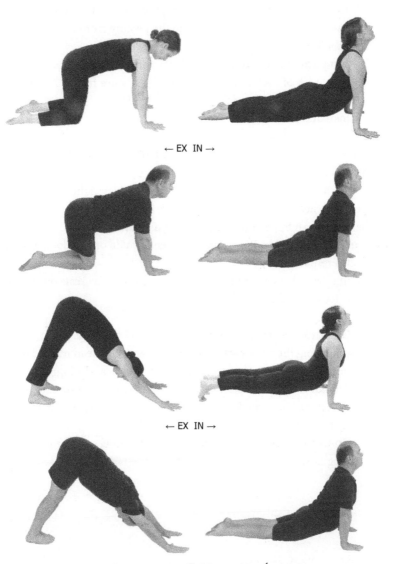

← EX   IN →

← EX   IN →

FIGURE 2.30 Upward Facing Dog (*Ūrdvha Mukha Śvānāsana*)

Sanskrit Name: *Ūrdhva Mukha Śvānāsana* [ˈurd hvʌ - ˈmʊk hʌ - ʃva ˈna sʌ nʌ]

Category: Symmetrical Prone Backward Bend

For the Singer: Strengthens the shoulders and arms, expands the chest, works the muscles of the torso, especially the upper back, and strengthens the feet, legs, and abdominal muscles

Difficulty Level: Intermediate

Classic Form: Arms are straight over hands placed beside hips, torso and head raised and pushed as far back as possible, legs stretched straight and not touching the floor, entire body resting on hands and tops of feet; come into the posture from the prone position

***Viniyoga* Adaptations:** Hands are more forward, legs may rest on floor, arch of back less deep; come into posture from a kneeling forward bend or from Downward Facing Dog

Instructions:

1) Begin either in a kneeling forward bend (Extended Child's Pose) or in Downward Facing Dog; exhale completely
2) Inhaling, stretch the body forward until arms are straight, supporting the upper body, arch the upper back, and look forward
3) Exhaling, return to position from which you started
4) If coming from Child's Pose, tops of the feet remain on the floor; lower legs may also remain on floor
5) If coming from Downward Facing Dog, the entire body rests on the hands and the toes turned under

Common Mistakes: Excessive arching of the lower back; collapsing the neck backward; leading with the head instead of initiating the movement with the back muscles; shrugging shoulders upward; rounding or hyperextending the shoulders

Risks: Strain to the lower back and neck muscles; compression of spinal discs; strain in the shoulders and wrists

Contraindications: Back injury; carpal tunnel syndrome; pregnancy

Supine

Axial Extension

♦ 31. Upward Feet Posture ⊙

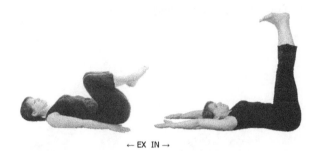

← EX IN →

FIGURE 2.31 Upward Feet Posture (*Ūrdhva Prasārita Pādāsana*)

Sanskrit Name: *Ūrdhva Prasārita Pādāsana* [ˈurd hvʌ -
prʌ ˈsa rɪ tʌ - pa ˈda sʌ nʌ]

Category: Symmetrical Supine Axial Extension with Forward
Bend

For the Singer: Extension of arms and legs in this posture flatten
cervical and lumbar curves of the spine and provide spinal
extension and excellent stretching for arms and legs

Difficulty Level: Beginning

Classic Form: Lying on back with arms stretched straight overhead
on floor, knees tightened, legs are lifted progressively to the
perpendicular position

***Viniyoga* Adaptations:** Posture begins with knees bent, feet off
floor, arms beside body; arms and legs are lifted simultaneously,
legs perpendicular or closer to torso, arms overhead on floor

Instructions:

1) Lie on back with arms beside torso, knees bent, feet off floor; exhale completely
2) Inhaling, tighten abdominal muscles and straighten legs upward, soles of
feet parallel to ceiling, and raise arms straight overhead to floor behind
head
3) Exhaling, bend knees to chest and return arms to floor beside torso

Common Mistakes: Failure to contract abdominal muscles before straightening legs and arms; legs come apart
Risks: Possible lower back strain if done improperly
Contraindications: Lower back injury

♦♦ 32. Supine Big Toe Holding Posture ⊙

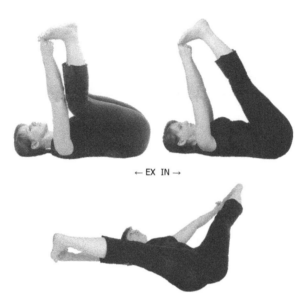

← EX IN →

FIGURE 2.32 Supine Big Toe Holding Posture (*Supta Prasārita Pādāṅguṣṭhāsana*)

Sanskrit Name: *Supta Prasārita Pādāṅguṣṭhāsana*
[ˈsʊp tʌ - prʌ ˈsa rɪ tʌ - ˈpa daŋ gʊʃt ˈha sʌ nʌ]
Category: Symmetrical Supine Extension Posture with Fixed Frame Forward Bend Component
For the Singer: Strong stretch of muscles of lower back, backs of legs, and inner thighs
Difficulty Level: Intermediate
Classic Form: Lying on back, hands holding big toes, legs perpendicular or closer to torso and then spread as wide apart as possible
Viniyoga **Adaptations:** Hands behind thighs just above the knee
Instructions:

1) Lying on back, inhale, exhaling, bend knees to chest and grasp big toes with hands
2) Inhaling, keeping shoulder blades on floor as much as possible, stretch heels upward, straightening legs
3) Exhale in position
4) Inhaling, open legs wide
5) Exhaling, close legs slowly; bend knees back to chest and release toes
6) Inhaling, return feet and arms to floor

> **Common Mistakes:** Allowing shoulders or sacrum to lift off floor, or chin to lift
> **Risks:** Overstretching shoulder girdle
> **Contraindications:** Shoulder or lower back injury

♦♦ 33. Tank ▶

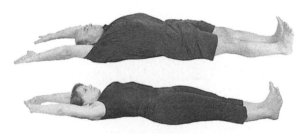

FIGURE 2.33   Tank (*Tāḍākamudrā*)

> **Sanskrit Name:** *Tāḍākamudrā* [ta da kʌ ˈmʊ dra]
> **Category:** Symmetrical Supine Extension Posture
> **For the Singer:** A strong spinal extension posture with a suspended breath component that greatly strengthens the abdominals and intercostals
> **Difficulty Level:** Intermediate
> **Classic Form:** Lying flat on back, legs stretched out, heels pushed out, arms stretched strongly overhead, hands clasped and turned outward
> ***Viniyoga* Adaptations:** Incorporation of a breath component—on exhale, the chest is expanded and lifted while the abdominals are pulled in and up; breath is suspended as whole body is stretched; hands may remain unclasped

Instructions:

1) Lying flat on the back, inhale and stretch arms overhead to the floor behind the head; clasp hands and turn hands outward or leave hands unclasped; push heels out
2) Exhaling, expand and lift the chest, pull abdominal muscles as high into the chest cavity as possible, stretch arms and hands overhead, and suspend breath with lungs empty
3) Inhaling, relax contracted muscles, and repeat, or unclasp hands and return arms to floor beside torso

> **Common Mistakes:** Overstretching the wrists or shoulders
> **Risks:** Stress to the wrists
> **Contraindications:** Wrist injury; pregnancy; acid reflux

♦ **34. Corpse** ⊙

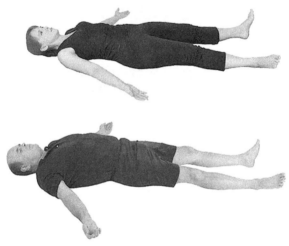

FIGURE 2.34 Corpse (*Śavāsana*)

Sanskrit Name: *Śavāsana* [ʃʌ ˈva sʌ nʌ]
Category: Supine Resting Posture
For the Singer: Posture for deep relaxation
Difficulty Level: Beginning
Classic Form: Lying flat on back, heels together, toes apart, arms on floor a little away from body, palms up; eyes closed; body relaxed; mind relaxed but alert to sensations in the body

***Viniyoga* Adaptations:** Feet a little apart
Instructions:

1) Lie flat on back, legs straight and a little apart, arms a little away from thighs, palms up
2) Close eyes, relax all muscles, and breathe deeply

> **Common Mistakes:** Legs bent; palms down; head turned to one side
> **Risks:** None, unless there are lower back problems

♦ **35. Supine Bound Angle** ⊙

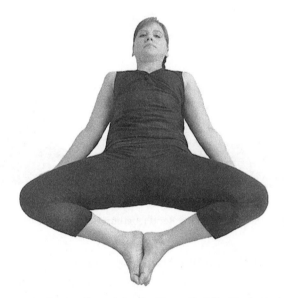

FIGURE 2.35 Supine Bound Angle (*Supta Baddha Koṇāsana*)

Sanskrit Name: *Supta Baddha Koṇāsana* [ˈsʊp tʌ - ˈbʌdːd hʌ - ko ˈna sʌ nʌ]
Category: Symmetrical Supine Extension Posture
For the Singer: Strongly stretches the inner thigh and groin muscles
Difficulty Level: Beginning
Classic Form: Lying on back, soles of feet together, knees on floor, arms on floor beside torso

Viniyoga **Adaptations:** Knees as far open as comfortable
Instructions:

1) Lying on back, arms by sides, knees bent, feet near buttocks; exhale
completely
2) Inhaling, open legs wide, putting soles of feet together
3) Exhaling, close legs very slowly

Common Mistakes: Feet too far away from buttocks; closing legs
quickly
Risks: Possible stress in hips or ankles
Contraindications: Knee, ankle, lower back, or hip injury

Forward Bends

♦ 36. Supine Forward Bend

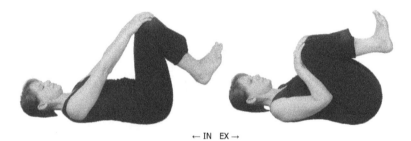

← IN   EX →

FIGURE 2.36 Supine Forward Bend (*Apānāsana*)

Sanskrit Name: *Apānāsana* [ʌ pa ˈna sʌ nʌ]
Category: Symmetrical or Asymmetrical Supine Forward Bend
For the Singer: A safe and effective stretch for the lower back
without bearing the weight of the chest, as in standing or kneeling
forward bends; a gentle massage of the internal organs
Difficulty Level: Beginning
Classic Form: Knees bent, knees and feet together, thighs close to
chest, hands on knees
Viniyoga **Adaptations:** Knees slightly apart to assist hip action
Instructions:

1) Lying on back, inhale, bend knees and lift feet off floor, hands straight on
knees, shoulder blades and head on floor

2) Exhaling, contract abdominal muscles and pull knees toward chest, flattening lumbar arch on floor, tuck chin

3) Inhaling, pull knees away from chest until arms are straight, allowing lumbar spine to arch again; chin remains tucked and shoulders on floor

> **Common Mistakes:** Lifting sacrum off floor; knees coming apart; lifting chin or shoulders
> **Risks:** Stress in lower back or sacroiliac joints; compression in hip joints or neck
> **Contraindications:** Severe lower back muscular or disc injury

Backward Bends

♦ 37. Bridge or Two-Footed Posture ▶

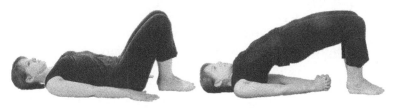

← EX IN →

FIGURE 2.37 Bridge or Two-Footed Posture (*Dvipāda Pīṭham*)

> **Sanskrit Name:** *Dvipāda Pīṭham* [dvɪ ˈpa dʌ - ˈpit hʌm]
> **Category:** Symmetrical Supine Backward Bend
> **For the Singer:** Deep stretching of the muscles of the chest and of the quadriceps; strong work in the hamstrings, gluteus, and upper spinal muscles; back of neck is also stretched
> **Difficulty Level:** Beginning
> **Classic Form:** Feet flat on floor, together or hip distance apart, as close to sit bones as possible; hands hold ankles; pelvis raised to high arch; neck and head remain on floor
> ***Viniyoga* Adaptations:** Feet farther away from sit bones; arms at sides; widen feet for greater hip opening

Instructions:

1) Lying on back, place feet flat on floor as close to sit bones as comfortable, arms at sides, palms down; exhale completely, contracting abdominals
2) Inhaling, press down with feet and lift pelvis off floor, tucking chin, pulling shoulder blades together, and lifting pelvis higher
3) Exhaling, contract abdominal muscles and slowly lower torso to floor, rolling down from top of spine one vertebra at a time (put shoulder blades down first)

Arm adaptations: on inhalation, raise arms one at a time or together overhead to the floor behind the head

Common Mistakes: Not lifting pelvis high enough; lifting chin; shifting weight to balls of feet, lifting heels
Risks: Compression in lower back either lifting or coming down; shear stress in knees; neck or shoulder strain
Contraindications: Neck, back, or knee injury

Lateral Bends

♦ 38. Supine Lateral Bend ▶

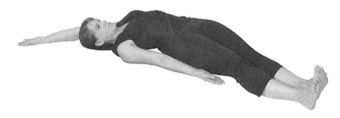

FIGURE 2.38 Supine Lateral Bend (*Jaṭhara Parivṛtti*, Lateral Variation)

Sanskrit Name: *Jaṭhara Parivṛtti*, Lateral
Variation [ˈdʒʌt hʌ rʌ - pʌ rɪ ˈvrt: tɪ]
Category: Asymmetrical Supine Lateral Bend
For the Singer: Gently stretches the entire torso, one side at a time; especially good stretch for the hip and rib cage muscles
Difficulty Level: Beginning
Classic Form: Usually performed as a standing posture with arms overhead, hands clasped, index fingers pointing upward

Viniyoga **Adaptations:** Use of the supine position and stretching one arm at a time overhead on the floor

Instructions:

1) Lie flat on the back, feet and legs together, arms a little away from torso
2) Keeping hips in place, walk both heels in small increments to one side until the opposite side of hips and lower torso are gently stretched; push heels out for stronger stretch; exhale completely
3) Inhaling, move arm on side of stretch along the floor until it is overhead, palm up
4) Stay in posture for several breaths, pushing heels out on inhale and relaxing on exhale
5) Exhaling, return arm to side; slowly walk heels back to center
6) Repeat on opposite side

Common Mistakes: Allowing hips to shift in the direction of the bend; overarching lower back; hyperextending the shoulder

Risks: Compression of spine if feet walk too far to one side; muscle strain in hips for same reason

Contraindications: Hip, shoulder, or spinal injury

Twists

♦ 39. Supine Abdominal Twist ▶

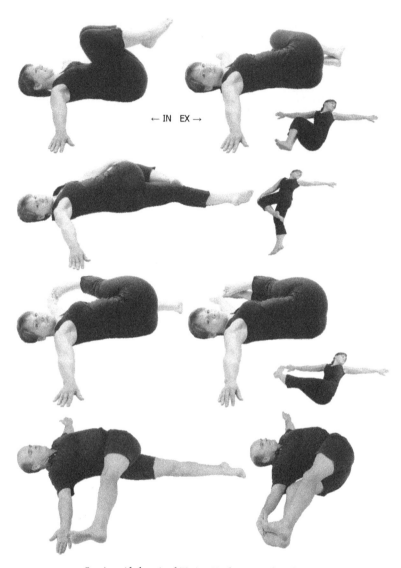

← IN   EX →

FIGURE 2.39 Supine Abdominal Twist (*Jaṭhara Parivṛtti*)

Sanskrit Name: *Jaṭhara Parivṛtti* [ˈdʒʌt hʌ rʌ - pʌ rɪ ˈvrt: tɪ]
Category: Supine Twist
For the Singer: Gently compresses the belly, stretches hip and neck muscles; useful for increasing length of exhalation; has many adaptations of legs that vary the intensity of the twist
Difficulty Level: Beginning
Classic Form: Legs are straight and lowered to the floor on one side together, toes close to hand; arms flat on floor at 90 degree angle to torso; abdomen rotated and head turned in opposite direction of legs
***Viniyoga* Adaptations:** Both knees bent toward chest before lowering both to side; one leg straight on floor, other leg bent or straight and lowered to floor on opposite side; straighten legs after bent knees reach the floor; arms on floor at or less than 90 degree angle
Instructions:

1) Lie flat on floor with arms out at 90 degree angle or less, palms down
2) Exhaling, bring feet off floor and knees to chest; inhale
3) Exhaling, contract lowest abdominal muscles to initiate twist and slowly lower bent knees (at 90 degree angle or less with chest) to the floor on one side, turning head in opposite direction, keeping opposite shoulder on or close to floor
4) Inhaling, lifting with the lower leg, return knees slowly to center
5) Repeat to opposite side

Leg adaptations: One or both legs straightened after twist, bringing foot or feet toward opposite hand; one leg straight on floor, bent knee of other leg lowered over straight leg; one leg straight on floor, other leg straight up and lowered across, bringing foot to or near opposite hand

Common Mistakes: Failing to initiate twist with lowest abdominal muscles; allowing opposite shoulder to rise off floor
Risks: Compression in lower back; stress in shoulder opposite direction of twist if shoulder muscles are tight; overstretching of hip muscles if tight
Contraindications: Lower back, hip, or shoulder injury

Seated

Axial Extension

♦♦ 40. Hero ⊙

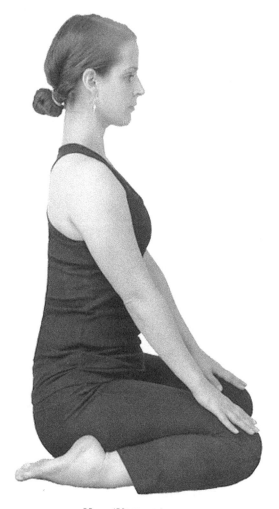

FIGURE 2.40 Hero (*Vīrāsana*)

Sanskrit Name: *Vīrāsana* [vi ˈra sʌ nʌ]
Category: Seated Posture
For the Singer: Deep stretching of the quadriceps and tops of the
ankles; also a spinal extension posture
Difficulty Level: Intermediate

Classic Form: Seated with legs folded back, knees together, feet spread apart resting on the floor outside of thighs, soles up and toes pointing straight back; wrists rest on knees, palms turned upward; spine erect

***Viniyoga* Adaptations:** Elbows bent, hands resting in lap for a more relaxed posture

Instructions:

1) Kneeling on floor, keeping knees together, spread feet a little over hip width apart
2) Sit down between the feet, buttocks resting on floor, feet at the sides of thighs, toes pointing straight back
3) Straighten spine, pull head a little back, chin a little down, extend arms until backs of wrists rest on knees for a good stretch (relax hands in lap for a more relaxed position)

> **Common Mistakes:** Sitting on feet instead of on floor
> **Risks:** Stress in ankles, tops of feet, or front of thighs
> **Contraindications:** Knee or ankle injury; tight quadriceps

♦ **41. Easy Seated Posture** ▶

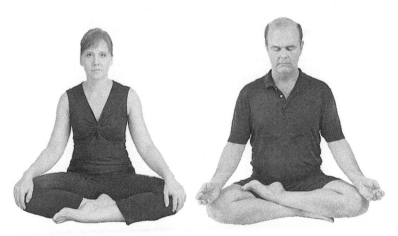

FIGURE **2.41** Easy Seated Posture (*Sukhāsana*)

Sanskrit Name: *Sukhāsana* [sʊk ˈha sʌ nʌ]
Category: Seated Extension Posture

For the Singer: An easy seated posture for *prāṇāyāma* or meditation; also functions as a spinal extension posture and for hip opening

Difficulty Level: Beginning

Classic Form: Sitting with legs crossed, tops of feet on floor, spine straight, head a little back, chin a little down, shoulders relaxed, hands on knees

***Viniyoga* Adaptations:** None (instead of crossing ankles, may fold one leg in until heel is at perineum and fold other leg in so that heels align, tops of feet on floor)

Instructions:

1) Sit on sit bones with legs stretched out on floor
2) Bend right knee and bring heel close to perineum, top of foot on floor
3) Bend left knee and bring heel in alignment with other heel, top of foot on floor; bring left foot to top of right calf if desired
4) Straighten spine, pull head a little back, chin a little down, and rest hands on knees or in lap

Common Mistakes: Resting sides of feet on floor; collapsing chest over belly; slumping shoulders; dropping head forward

Risks: Stress in hips or knees because of outward rotation; stress in ankles

Contraindications: Knee, hip, or ankle injury

♦♦ 42. Stick or Staff Posture ▶

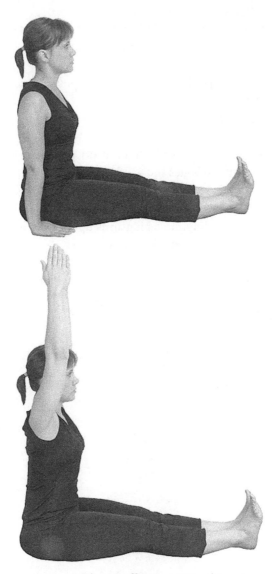

FIGURE 2.42 Stick or Staff Posture (*Daṇḍāsana*)

Sanskrit Name: *Daṇḍāsana* [dʌn ˈda sʌ nʌ]
Category: Seated Extension Posture

For the Singer: A strong stretch for the entire back, shoulder girdle, arms, and legs; strengthens all postural muscles

Difficulty Level: Intermediate

Classic Form: Seated with legs straight out, knees on floor, spine erect, arms overhead, elbows straight, hands clasped and turned to ceiling

Viniyoga Adaptations: Knees very slightly bent to avoid lower back strain

Instructions:

1) Sitting with legs straight out in front at 90 degrees to the torso, bring weight of torso onto sit bones and hands to floor beside hips, arms straight; exhale completely
2) Inhaling, lift chest away from belly, raise arms overhead, clasp hands and turn palms toward ceiling, stretching arms upward and heels forward
3) Exhaling, lower arms and relax knees and ankles

Common Mistakes: Rotating pelvis too far forward; overstretching shoulder muscles; collapsing chest over belly

Risks: Compression or muscle strain in the lower back; strain in the shoulders

Contraindications: Lower back or shoulder injury

♦♦ 43. Bound Angle ▶

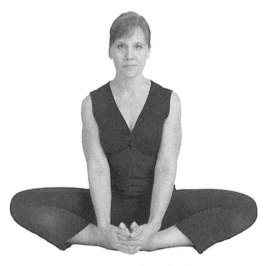

FIGURE 2.43 Bound Angle (*Baddha Koṇāsana*)

Sanskrit Name: *Baddha Koṇāsana* [ˈbʌdːd hʌ - ko ˈna sʌ nʌ]
For the Singer: A challenging spinal extension posture; strongly stretches inner thigh and groin muscles; creates circulation in pelvic area
Difficulty Level: Intermediate
Classic Form: Sitting with soles of feet together, heels touching perineum, knees on or toward floor, hands grasping feet, stretch spine erect
***Viniyoga* Adaptations:** None
Instructions:

1) Sitting with legs stretched straight out, bend knees and bring feet close to torso
2) Bring soles of feet together, heels touching perineum
3) Widen legs until knees rest on or close to floor
4) Grasp feet with hands and stretch spine upward, head a little back, chin a little down

Common Mistakes: Heels not at perineum; collapsing chest over belly; jutting chin forward
Risks: Stress in knees, hips, or ankles
Contraindications: Knee, hip, or ankle injury

Forward Bends

♦ 44. Seated Forward Bend ▶

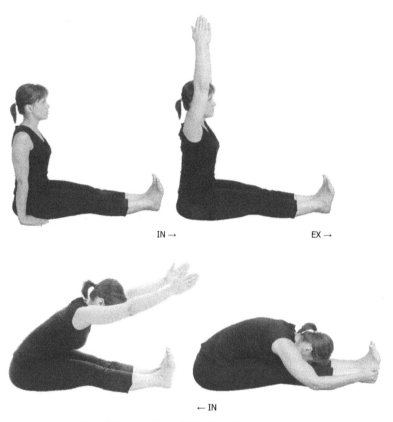

IN →   EX →

← IN

FIGURE 2.44 Seated Forward Bend (*Paścimatānāsana*)

Sanskrit Name: *Paścimatānāsana* [ˈpʌʃ tʃɪ mʌ ta ˈna sʌ nʌ]
Category: Symmetrical Seated Forward Bend
For the Singer: A deep stretch for the muscles of the lower back;
all major abdominal and trunk flexor muscles are worked; extensor
muscles of the spine and the shoulder girdle muscles are worked in
return to upright position; secondary hamstring stretch
Difficulty Level: Beginning
Classic Form: Legs straight, feet together, hands holding feet, head
on legs beyond knees
***Viniyoga* Adaptations:** Slightly bent knees; feet slightly apart
Instructions:

1) Sitting with feet slightly apart, rotate pelvis forward to place torso weight on sit bones; exhale completely
2) Inhaling, lift chest up from belly, raise arms overhead, tuck chin
3) Exhaling, contract lowest abdominal muscles to initiate bend forward; slightly bend knees and continue contracting abdominals while bringing belly toward thighs, keeping upper back flat, head and arms aligned
4) Inhaling, abdominals remaining contracted, pull chest and arms forward and up, keeping upper back flat, head and arms aligned
5) Exhaling, lower arms

> **Common Mistakes:** Weight not on sit bones; bending from hips causing too much pelvic rotation; keeping knees locked; collapsing chest over belly; rotation of knees; jutting chin
> **Risks:** Compression or muscle strain in lower back; stress in sacrum or sacroiliac joints; strain in neck and shoulder girdle muscles
> **Contraindications:** Back or shoulder injury

♦ **45. Boat** ▶

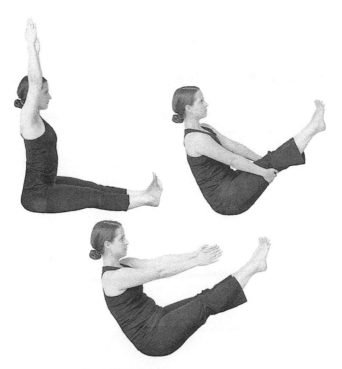

FIGURE 2.45 Boat (*Nāvāsana*)

Sanskrit Name: *Nāvāsana* [na ˈva sʌ nʌ]
Category: Seated Balanced Forward Bend
For the Singer: Greatly strengthens the abdominal and lower back muscles
Difficulty Level: Beginning
Classic Form: Whole body balanced on sit bones with raised torso and legs forming an obtuse angle (greater than 90 degrees); legs and arms together and straight, toes at eye level, palms together, chin tucked in
Viniyoga Adaptations: Allow lower back to round slightly, transferring more work to the abdominal muscles; may begin with a smaller angle
Instructions:

1) Sit with legs straight and together, hands on floor beside hips; exhale completely
2) Inhaling, lift chest away from belly, raise arms overhead, tuck chin
3) Exhaling, slightly tilt pelvis backward and slightly round lower back; contract abdominal muscles strongly and lean torso back as legs are lifted and arms brought forward parallel to the floor, palms together or facing each other, chin tucked in, toes at eye level
4) Inhaling, return to seated position

Common Mistakes: Too much rounding of lower back; collapsing chest over belly; jutting chin forward
Risks: Compression and muscle strain in lower back; tension in neck and shoulders
Contraindications: Neck or lower back injury

♦ **46. Seated Triangle** ▶

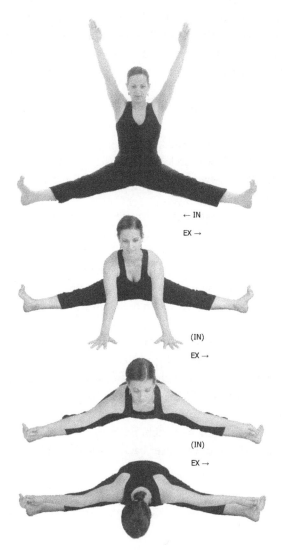

← IN

EX →

(IN)

EX →

(IN)

EX →

FIGURE 2.46 Seated Triangle (*Upaviṣṭha Koṇāsana*)

Sanskrit Name: *Upaviṣṭha Koṇāsana* [ʊ pʌ ˈvɪʃt hʌ -
ko ˈna sʌ nʌ]
Category: Seated Forward Bend with Spread Legs
For the Singer: Deep stretch in lower back, inner thighs, arms,
and shoulders

Difficulty Level: Beginning
Classic Form: Sitting with legs stretched out as wide as possible, torso is folded forward, hands grasp feet, chin on floor
***Viniyoga* Adaptations:** Knees slightly bent, torso folded forward, arms stretched out in front, forehead on or close to floor
Instructions:

1) Sitting with erect spine, legs spread wide, knees slightly bent, exhale completely
2) Inhaling, raise arms overhead
3) Exhaling, contract lower abdominal muscles and fold forward, bringing torso toward floor between legs, arms out in front or grasping feet, forehead toward or on floor
4) Inhaling, abdominals strongly contracted, pull chest and arms forward and up, leading with the chest, and return to upright position
5) Exhaling, lower arms; Variations: a) Exhale forward and grasp toes with hands; stay 2–4 breaths, lifting chest on inhale and folding farther forward on exhale; arms can be used for leverage; b) Rotate torso to face one leg; exhale forward and grasp foot with both hands; repeat to opposite side

Common Mistakes: Too much forward rotation of pelvis; collapsing chest over belly; not leading with chest to return to upright, placing too much stress on lower back; jutting chin forward; rotation of hips, knees, and feet
Risks: Muscle strain in lower back and hip joints; shoulder girdle strain in returning to upright position
Contraindications: Lower back or shoulder injury

◆ ◆ **47. Head to Knee Posture** ▶

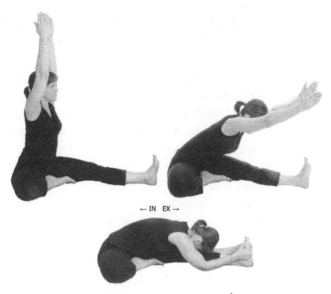

← IN EX →

FIGURE **2.47** Head to Knee Posture (*Jānu Śirṣāsana*)

Sanskrit Name: *Jānu Śirṣāsana* [ˈdʒa nʊ - ʃɪr ˈʃas ʌ nʌ]
Category: Asymmetrical Seated Forward Bend
For the Singer: Stretches the lower back, one side at a time, as
well as the entire outstretched leg side of the body, including
hamstrings in the stay position when knee can be safely
straightened on inhale
Difficulty Level: Intermediate
Classic Form: Seated with straight spine, one leg straight out in
front, back of knee on floor, the other bent on the floor at a wide
angle so that the knee is as far back as possible, heel to groin, with
toes touching the opposite inner thigh; both hands grasp toes of
outstretched leg; torso is pulled forward over the thigh; head rests
on or below knee
Viniyoga **Adaptations:** Knee of bent leg at right angle to hip, heel
to groin, sole of foot against opposite inner thigh; arm on side of
straight leg folded behind back, opposite arm straight up; in the
forward bend, the hand opposite the straight leg grasps toes (or
both arms may be used together)

Instructions:

1) Seated erect with legs stretched straight out in front, bend one knee and bring the heel of the foot to the groin and the sole to the opposite thigh, leaving the side of foot and leg on floor; fold arm behind back; exhale completely
2) Inhaling, raise arm on side of bent knee straight overhead, lifting the chest away from the solar plexus and slightly tucking the chin
3) Exhaling, contract the abdominals, keeping the upper back flat and slightly bending the outstretched knee, fold forward, bringing belly and chest to thigh and hand to toes of outstretched leg
4) Inhaling, keeping abdominal muscles contracted, pull chest forward and up, releasing toes, and return to upright position
5) Exhaling, lower arm(s)
6) Repeat on opposite side; Variation: Use both arms

Common Mistakes: Collapsing chest over belly; leaving abdominal muscles slack; raising chin and compressing neck; executing bend with straight knee, risking overstretching the lower back

Risks: Stress in lower back

Contraindications: Knee, back, or shoulder injury

Backward Bends

♦♦♦ **48. Supine Hero** ▶

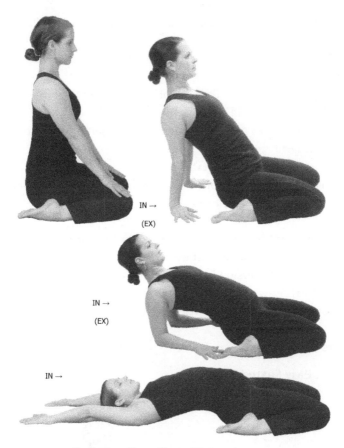

FIGURE 2.48 Supine Hero (*Supta Vīrāsana*)

Sanskrit Name: *Supta Vīrāsana* [ˈsʊp tʌ - vi ˈra sʌ nʌ]
Category: Seated Backward Bend
For the Singer: Deep stretch for the front of the thighs, pelvic region, abdomen, and chest; also for arms and shoulders; deep arch of back
Difficulty Level: Advanced
Classic Form: Reclining with legs folded back as in *Vīrāsana*, torso and head on floor, arms overhead on floor behind head

Viniyoga Adaptations: Arms may remain on floor beside torso
Instructions:

1) Sitting in *Vīrāsana,* exhale completely
2) Inhaling, recline the torso back and rest the elbows on the floor, one at a time; exhale
3) Inhaling, rest the top of the head on the floor, extending arms forward; exhale
4) Inhaling, gradually lower the back of the head and then the torso to the floor; the lower back will arch; exhale
5) Inhaling, raise arms and stretch them out straight overhead on the floor behind the head
6) Stay in posture for several breaths
7) Exhaling, return arms to floor beside torso; inhaling, lift torso up on elbows, and exhaling return to *Vīrāsana*

> **Common Mistakes:** Sitting on feet in *Vīrāsana*; moving too quickly into or out of posture
> **Risks:** Compression in lower back; stress in thighs, ankles, or tops of feet
> **Contraindications:** Lower back, knee, or ankle injury

Twists

♦ 49. Easy Seated Twist ▶

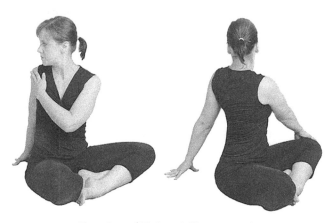

FIGURE 2.49 Easy Seated Twist (*Sukhāsana Parivṛtti*)

Sanskrit Name: *Sukhāsana Parivṛtti* [sʊk 'ha sʌ nʌ -
pʌ rɪ 'vrt: tɪ]
Category: Seated Twisting Posture
For the Singer: Rotates spine, building strength and flexibility in
the spinal muscles; stretches the muscles of the rib cage
Difficulty Level: Beginning
Classic Form: Seated cross legged with extended spine, one hand
on floor behind back, other hand on opposite shoulder, head turned
to look backward over shoulder
***Viniyoga* Adaptations:** Use of breath patterns for tension and
release
Instructions:

1) Sit in *Sukhāsana*; exhale completely
2) Inhaling, lift and expand chest, extending spine upward, head a little back,
   chin a little down
3) Exhaling, strongly contract abdominal muscles and twist upper torso to
   one side, placing hand on side of twist on the floor behind back and other
   hand on opposite shoulder; turn head to look over shoulder
4) Inhaling, extend spine
5) Exhaling, deepen twist
6) Inhaling, turn head, then shoulders forward, releasing hands and returning to *Sukhāsana*
7) Repeat to opposite side

> **Common Mistakes:** Collapsing chest over belly; jutting chin
> forward; tightening jaw and/or shoulders
> **Risks:** Overrotating the spine; stress in shoulders or hips
> **Contraindications:** Spinal injury

♦ ♦ **50. Half Seated Twist** ▶

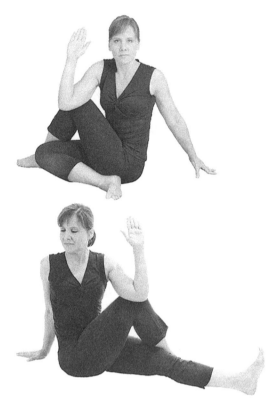

FIGURE 2.50 Half Seated Twist (*Ardha Matsyendrāsana*)

Sanskrit Name: *Ardha Matsyendrāsana* [ˈʌrd hʌ - mʌ tsjen ˈdra sʌ nʌ]

Category: Seated Twisting Posture

For the Singer: Rotates spine, building strength and flexibility in the spinal muscles; stretches the muscles of the rib cage; a deeper twist than *Sukhāsana Parivṛtti*

Difficulty Level: Intermediate

Classic Form: One leg bent so that the buttocks rest on the foot; other leg crossed over bent leg so that the foot rests on the floor on the outside of the opposite thigh; torso turned 90 degrees until upright knee can slip under opposite armpit; other hand reaches around behind back until hands can be clasped to the side

Viniyoga **Adaptations:** Foot of bent leg remains on floor beside hip, rather than underneath buttocks; hand on the side of the twist rests on the floor behind the back; opposite arm wraps around upright knee, palm resting on hip or upper thigh, or elbow outside upright knee, palm facing outward

Instructions:

1) Sit with left leg folded on floor, foot beside right hip and cross right foot over to outside of left knee (may be done with straight leg)
2) Inhaling, lift chest and straighten spine
3) Exhaling, place right hand on floor behind back and left arm on outside of right thigh, elbow outside the knee, and left hand at hip, or hand raised with palm facing outward
4) Inhaling, lift chest and extend spine more
5) Exhaling, strongly contract lowest abdominal muscles, twist torso to the right, and look over right shoulder
6) Stay in position several breaths; inhaling, relax twist and extend spine, exhaling, deepen twist using arms for leverage
7) Inhaling, turn head, then shoulders forward, releasing arms, and returning to forward facing position
8) Repeat to opposite side

Common Mistakes: Initiating twist with shoulders instead of lowest abdominal muscles; collapsing chest over belly; jutting chin forward; overrotating spine; displacing hips in direction of twist

Risks: Compression of spinal discs; stress in sacroiliac, hip, and knee joints

Contraindications: Spinal disc injury, lower back, hip, or knee injury

Lateral/Twist

♦♦♦ 51. Revolved Head to Knee ▶

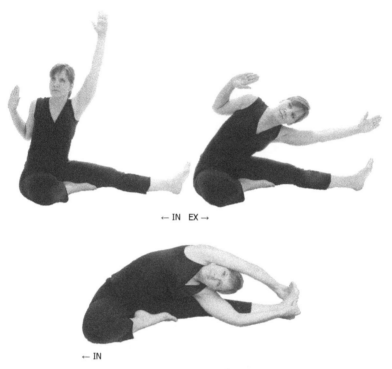

← IN   EX →

← IN

FIGURE 2.51 Revolved Head to Knee (*Jānu Śirṣāsana Parivṛtti*)

Sanskrit Name: *Jānu Śirṣāsana Parivṛtti* [ˈdʒa nʊ - ʃɪr ˈʃa sʌ nʌ - pʌ rɪ ˈvrːt tɪ]

Category: Asymmetrical Seated Lateral Bend with Twist

For the Singer: A challenging, invigorating posture that stretches the sides of the body while rotating the spine at the same time; excellent for flexibility in lower back, hips, and shoulders

Difficulty Level: Advanced

Classic Form: Seated in *Jānu Śirṣāsana*, the hand on the side of the extended leg grasps the inside of the foot, the torso is folded laterally over the leg and rotated as far as possible to the outside with the opposite arm reaching overhead to grasp the foot on the outside; the head rests on the knee

***Viniyoga* Adaptations:** Extended leg is at an angle away from the midline; knee of extended leg is slightly bent

Instructions:

1) Sitting with legs extended, fold right leg in, heel to groin, and shift the left leg outward at a slight angle; exhale completely
2) Inhaling, raise left arm straight up and right arm up with elbow bent; turn shoulders to the right, aligned with extended leg
3) Exhaling, contract lower abdominal muscles, bend left knee slightly, and bend laterally to the left, bringing left hand to inside of left foot, thumb pointing downward, and left side of torso to leg
4) Inhaling, extend right arm forward over head, stretching right side of torso
5) Exhaling, bend closer to leg
6) Inhaling, bring right hand to left foot and rotate chest upward so that shoulders are aligned vertically; exhale
7) Inhaling, release hands and return to upright position
8) Exhaling, lower arms
9) Repeat on opposite side

> **Common Mistakes:** Initiating twist at shoulders rather than with deep abdominal muscles; displacing hips in direction of twist; collapsing chest over belly
>
> **Risks:** Compression in spine; stress in hips, shoulders, and neck
>
> **Contraindications:** Spine, shoulder, hip, or neck injury

Inversions

♦♦ **52. Inverted Posture** ▶

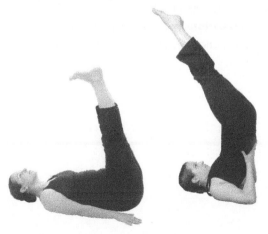

← EX   IN →

FIGURE 2.52 Inverted Posture (*Viparīta Karaṇī*)

Sanskrit Name: *Viparīta Karaṇī* [vɪ pʌ ˈri tʌ - kʌ rʌ ˈni]

Category: Inversion

For the Singer: The benefits of turning the body upside down on the internal organs—reversing the pull of gravity and revitalizing the organs (*viparīta*—active reversal); strengthens the entire musculature of the torso

Difficulty Level: Intermediate

Classic Form: With the body resting on shoulders, neck, and back of head, the spine and legs are held in vertical alignment, the hands at the waist supporting the hips

***Viniyoga* Adaptations:** Legs may be held at a slight angle rather than vertically

Instructions:

1) Lying on back, inhale; contract lowest abdominal muscles
2) Exhaling, flip or raise legs (knees bent or straight) up overhead, lifting buttocks and mid-back off floor, supporting hips with hands at waist (straighten bent knees); press shoulders and upper arms into floor
3) Take several breaths in the position
4) Exhaling, bend knees toward chest
5) Inhaling, return to lying flat on floor

Common Mistakes: Performing inversion without proper preparation; failing to press shulders and upper arms into floor to relieve neck of entire body weight

Risks: Compression of vertebrae in the neck or lower back; stress in the shoulders and neck

Contraindications: Headache; high blood pressure; back or neck injury; pregnancy; menstruation; heavy lower torso (obesity); retinal detachment

♦ 53. Legs up the Wall Posture ▶

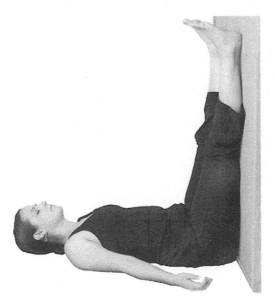

FIGURE 2.53 Legs up the Wall Posture

Sanskrit Name: *Viparīta Karaṇī*, Supported
Variation vɪ pʌ ˈri tʌ - kʌ rʌ ˈni
Category: Inversion (Supported Half Inversion)
For the Singer: Legs up the Wall provides a simple and relaxing way to restore circulation to the legs after air travel or after long periods of standing; other benefits include relaxing the whole torso, opening the front of the torso, relieving various conditions related to emotional states
Difficulty Level: Beginning
Instructions:

1) Placing a bolster or folded blanket for support of the pelvis a few inches away from a wall, sit on the support parallel to the wall and, exhaling, smoothly swing legs up against the wall and torso gently onto the floor perpendicular to wall

2) Bring the sit bones close to the wall, and adjust the support until the front of your torso arches gently; place a folded cloth under the neck if the neck is too flat on the floor; relax arms out to sides, palms up

3) Keep legs just firm enough to stay vertical on the wall

4) Remain in posture 5—15 minutes
5) Remove support before inhaling out of posture to avoid twisting as you come back to a sitting position

> **Common Mistakes:** Sit bones either too close to or too far away from the wall
> **Risks:** Coming into and out of the posture can strain the lower back if done improperly
> **Contraindications:** Yoga teachers are divided on whether this posture should be done during menstruation. It should be avoided by those with serious eye or neck problems.

♦♦♦ **54. Shoulderstand**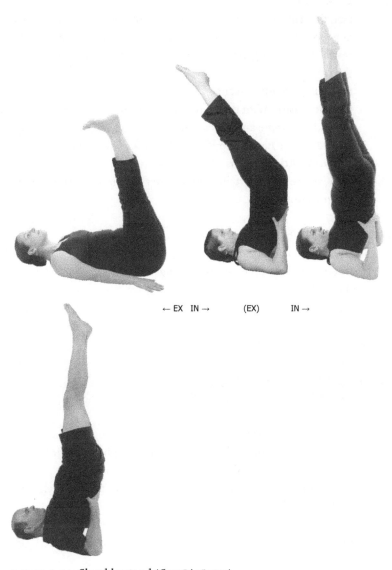

← EX IN →   (EX)   IN →

FIGURE 2.54 Shoulderstand (*Sarvāṅgāsana*)

Sanskrit Name: *Sarvāṅgāsana* [sʌr vaŋ ˈga sʌ nʌ]
Category: Inversion
For the Singer: Provides the benefits of turning the body upside down on the internal organs—reversing the pull of gravity and revitalizing the organs; strengthens the entire musculature of the torso
Difficulty Level: Advanced
Classic Form: With the body resting on shoulders, neck, and back of head, the spine and legs are held in vertical alignment above the shoulders, the hands supporting the back above the waist
***Viniyoga* Adaptations:** In full posture, legs are held at a slight angle to the pelvis, avoiding excessive strain in the lumbar spine
Instructions:

1) Lying on back, inhale; contract lowest abdominal muscles
2) Exhaling, flip or raise legs up over head (knees may be bent initially), lifting buttocks and mid-back off floor, supporting mid-back with hands; straighten legs if knees bent
3) Inhaling, raise legs upward, hips vertically above elbows, toes over eyes, legs held at a slight angle to pelvis; press shoulders and upper arms into floor
4) Take several breaths in the position
5) Exhaling, bend knees toward chest
6) Inhaling, return to lying flat on floor
7) Turn over and do 2–4 repetitions of Cobra as compensation for this posture

Common Mistakes: Performing Shoulderstand without proper preparation; failing to press shoulders and upper arms into the floor to relieve the neck of the weight of the entire body
Risks: Compression of vertebrae in the neck or lower back; stress in the shoulders and neck
Contraindications: Headache; high blood pressure; back or neck injury; pregnancy; menstruation; heavy lower torso (obesity); retinal detachment
CAUTION: *This posture should not be attempted without first having personal instruction from a qualified teacher.* Do not perform Shoulderstand in isolation. Always place it in the middle of the proper sequence of preparatory and compensatory postures.

♦♦♦ 55. Plough ⊚

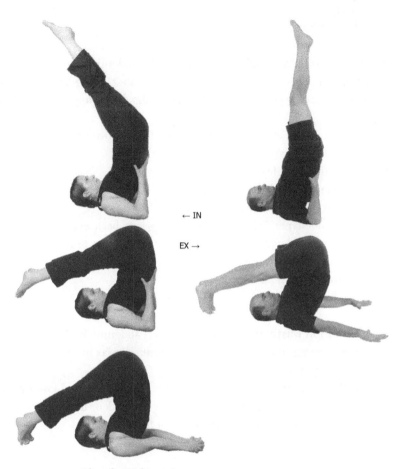

← IN

EX →

FIGURE 2.55 Plough (*Halāsana*)

Sanskrit Name: *Halāsana* [hʌ ˈla sʌ nʌ]
Category: Inverted Forward Bend [Forward Bend Variation of Shoulderstand]
For the Singer: Strengthens the entire back and torso; stretches legs and back; compresses internal organs
Difficulty Level: Advanced
Classic Form: From Shoulderstand, feet are dropped back over head, legs straight, back remains vertical, weight on shoulders, neck, and head; arms are straight on floor in opposite direction from legs, fingers interlaced

Viniyoga **Adaptations:** Back allowed to round slightly; hands hold feet, stretch out in opposite direction, or continue to support back

Instructions:

1) From lying flat on floor: inhale; contract lowest abdominal muscles
2) Exhaling and supporting the lower back with hands, bring knees to chest or forehead, back vertical to floor, weight on shoulders, upper arms, neck, and head
3) Inhaling straighten legs out and touch toes to floor overhead; continue to support back with hands
4) Stay in position for a few breaths
5) Exhaling, bend knees back to forehead
6) Inhaling, bring torso and feet back to floor, stretch out legs
7) From Shoulderstand: Exhaling, slowly drop legs back overhead, toes to floor, keeping hands on back for support or bend knees to forehead, then straighten legs to touch toes to floor behind head
8) Inhaling, return to Shoulderstand
9) Exhaling, bend knees to chest; inhaling, return torso to floor

Common Mistakes: Failing to contract abdominals before moving legs; leaving shoulder and upper arm muscles lax instead of pressing into the floor

Risks: Strain to the muscles of the neck, shoulders, and lower back

Contraindications: High blood pressure; back or neck injury; pregnancy; menstruation; heavy lower torso (obesity)

Face and Neck

♦♦ **56. Lion** ▷

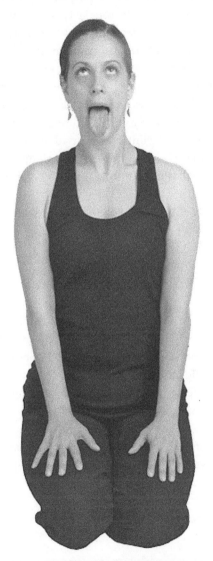

FIGURE 2.56 Lion (*Simhāsana*)

Sanskrit Name: *Simhāsana* [sɪm ˈha sʌ nʌ]
Category: Seated Tongue and Facial Stretch
For the Singer: Stretches the tongue, jaw, and facial muscles; also said to cure bad breath, cleanse the tongue, and contribute to clearer speech; works knees, ankles, abdominal muscles, chest muscles, fingers, and breathing mechanism
Difficulty Level: Intermediate
Classic Form: Sitting on crossed ankles under buttocks, spine straight, hands on knees, arms stretched stiff, fingers stretched apart, jaw open as wide as possible, tongue stretched out as far as possible (tip toward chin), eyes focused up to forehead or at tip of nose, exhaling "Haaah" forcefully through the mouth; may also be done in Lotus Posture, learning forward with hands on the floor, arms straight, fingers spread
Adaptation: Sit in simple Hero posture (without crossing ankles); can also be done sitting on a chair
Instructions:

1) Kneel and cross right ankle over left ankle and sit back on right heel (or sit in Hero posture)
2) Place hands firmly on knees, spreading fingers wide apart, arms straight
3) Open jaw and eyes wide, stretch tongue forward and down as far as possible, tip toward or touching chin; focus eyes at forehead or tip of nose
4) Inhale slowly through nose
5) Exhale slowly but forcefully through mouth, making a "Haaah" sound as air is felt coming over the back of the tongue
6) Stay in the posture for several breaths
7) Release from posture, cross left ankle over right ankle, and repeat the sequence (not necessary to repeat if using Hero posture)

Risks: Stress in knees and ankles
Contraindications: Knee or ankle injury (sit on a chair)

57. Eye Stretches

For the Singer: Strengthen eye muscles in all directions; helpful for quick visual shifts on stage

Instructions:

1) Sit or stand with erect spine and relaxed shoulders and keep head absolutely still; repeat each motion 5–10 times
2) Look as far up and as far down as possible
3) Look as far to the right and as far to the left as possible
4) Look as far up and right and as far down and left as possible
5) Look as far up and left and as far down and right as possible
6) Imagine a clock face as large in diameter as your outstretched arms; keeping head absolutely still, look at each number clockwise from 12 to 12, then counterclockwise, twice each
7) Place your thumb close to your face and look back and forth from thumb to far object 10 times, eyes separately and together
8) Rub palms together fast and hard until they are warm; place warm palms over closed eyes to rest the muscles

58. Neck Stretches

For the Singer: Stretch the neck muscles in all directions; helps to keep the neck supple for head rotation; relieves stiff neck muscles; may be done with a breathing pattern

Instructions:

1) Sit or stand with a straight spine and relaxed shoulders
2) Drop chin toward chest, stretching the back of the neck; repeat 2–4 times, then hold 2–4 breaths
3) Look up toward ceiling and stretch chin muscles; repeat 2–4 times, then hold 2–4 breaths
4) Bring right ear as close to right shoulder as possible; repeat 2–4 times, then hold 2–4 breaths; repeat on left side
5) Look as far over shoulder to the right as possible; repeat 2–4 times, then hold 2–4 breaths; repeat on left side
6) Repeat each direction once and hold a few seconds

Caution: Do not overstretch the neck, especially backward to avoid disc compression in the cervical spine.

Āsanas for Each Area

There are several physical postures (*āsanas*) of beginning and intermediate difficulty that are effective for each area of the body. Taking the order of the areas mentioned in the first part of the chapter, the following section lists a number of postures for each area from which various sequences can be constructed. The numbers refer to the Numbered List of *āsanas*. Sequences for each area are found in Part II: Practices for the Student.

Postural Muscles

Feet and Legs

1. Balanced Standing Posture (*Samasthiti*) [18] ▶
2. Mountain Posture (*Tāḍāsana*) with arm and heel raises [19–20] ▶
6. Chair Posture (*Utkatāsana*) [28] ▶
9. Warrior (*Vīrabhadrāsana*) [34] ▶
7. Intense Side Stretch (*Pārśvottānāsana*) [30] ▶
5. Spread Legs Forward Bend (*Prasārita Pādottānāsana*) [26] ▶
11. Extended Lateral Angle (*Utthita Pārśva Koṇāsana*) [38] ▶
10. Extended Triangle (*Utthita Trikoṇāsana*) [36] ▶
12. Revolved Triangle (*Trikoṇāsana Parivṛtti*) [40] ▶
47. Head to Knee (*Jānu Śirṣāsana*) [95] ▶

Lower Abdominal Muscles

4. Half Forward Bend (*Ardha Uttānāsana*) [24] ▶
8. Half Intense Side Stretch (*Ardha Pārśvottānāsana*) [32] ▶
25. Cobra (*Bhujaṅgāsana*) [64] ▶
26. Locust (*Śalabhāsana*) [65] ▶
27. Half Locust (*Ardha Śalabhāsana*) [67] ▶
28. Chariot or Airplane (*Vimānāsana*) [68] ▶
29. Bow (*Dhanurāsana*) [70] ▶
45. Boat (*Nāvāsana*) [91] ▶
54. Shoulderstand (*Sarvāṅgāsana*) [107] ▶

Lower Back

4. Half Forward Bend (*Ardha Uttānāsana*) [24] ▶
8. Half Intense Side Stretch (*Ardha Pārśvottānāsana*) [32] ▶
19. Ruddy Goose (*Cakravākāsana*) [53] ▶
36. Supine Forward Bend (*Apānāsana*) [78] ▶
31. Upward Feet Posture (*Ūrdhva Prasārita Pādāsana*) [73] ▶

37. Bridge or Two-Footed Posture (*Dvipāda Pīṭham*) [79] ⊙
44. Seated Forward Bend (*Paścimatānāsana*) [90] ⊙

Upper Back

2. Mountain Posture (*Tāḍāsana*) with arm raises [19–20] ⊙
9. Warrior (*Vīrhabdrāsana*) [34] ⊙
25. Cobra (*Bhujaṅgāsana*) [64] ⊙
27. Half Locust (*Ardha Śalabhāsana*) [67] ⊙
26. Locust (*Śalabhāsana*) [65] ⊙
46. Seated Triangle (*Upaviṣṭha Koṇāsana*) [93] ⊙

Shoulders and Neck

2. Mountain Posture (*Tāḍāsana*) with arm raises [19–20] ⊙
9. Warrior (*Vīrhabdrāsana*) with arm variations [34] ⊙
20. Kneeling Forward Bend (*Vajrāsana*) with head turns [55] ⊙
18. Downward Facing Dog (*Adho Mukha Śvānāsana*) [51] ⊙
30. Upward Facing Dog (*Ūrdvha Mukha Śvānāsana*) [71] ⊙
37. Bridge or Two-Footed Posture (*Dvipāda Pīṭham*) [79] ⊙
54. Shoulderstand (*Sarvāṅgāsana*) [107] ⊙
55. Plough (*Halāsana*) [109] ⊙

Spinal Extension

2. Mountain Posture (*Tāḍāsana*) with arm and heel raises [19–20] ⊙
18. Downward Facing Dog (*Adho Mukha Śvānāsana*) [51] ⊙
32. Supine Big Toe Holding Posture (*Supta Prasārita Pādāṅguṣṭhāsana*) [74] ⊙
42. Stick or Staff (*Daṇḍāsana*) [87] ⊙
33. Tank (*Tāḍākamudrā*) [75] ⊙
40. Hero (*Vīrāsana*) [84] ⊙
48. Supine Hero (*Supta Vīrāsana*) [97] ⊙
41. Easy Seated Posture (*Sukhāsana*) [85] ⊙
34. Corpse (*Śavāsana*) [76] ⊙

Movement Muscles and Joints

Feet and Legs

2. Mountain Posture (*Tāḍāsana*) with arm and heel raises [19–20] ⊙
9. Warrior (*Vīrhabdrāsana*) [34] ⊙
11. Extended Lateral Angle (*Utthita Pārśva Koṇāsana*) [38] ⊙

10. Extended Triangle (*Utthita Trikoṇāsana*) [36] ▶
47. Head to Knee (*Jānu Śirṣāsana*) [95] ▶

Hips

37. Bridge or Two-Footed Posture (*Dvipāda Pīṭham*) widening feet [79] ▶
35. Supine Bound Angle (*Supta Baddha Koṇāsana*) [77] ▶
32. Supine Big Toe Holding Posture (*Supta Prasārita Pādāṅguṣṭhāsana*) [74] ▶
43. Bound Angle (*Baddha Koṇāsana*) [88] ▶
46. Seated Triangle (*Upaviṣṭha Koṇāsana*) [93] ▶
21. One-Footed Pigeon King (*Ekapāda Rājakapotāsana*) with forward bend variation [57] ▶
22. Lizard (*Godhāpīṭham*) with forward bend variation [59] ▶

Spinal Flexibility

38. Supine Lateral Bend (*Jaṭhara Parivṛtti*, Lateral Variation) [80] ▶
12. Revolved Triangle (*Trikoṇāsana Parivṛtti*) [40] ▶
39. Supine Abdominal Twist (*Jaṭhara Parivṛtti*) [82] ▶
49. Easy Seated Posture with Twist (*Sukhāsana Parivṛtti*) [98] ▶
50. Half Seated Twist (*Ardha Matsyendrāsana*) [100] ▶
51. Revolved Head to Knee (*Jānu Śirṣāsana Parivṛtti*) [102] ▶

Arms, Shoulders, and Neck

57. Neck Stretches [113] <no video>
2. Mountain Posture (*Tāḍāsana*) with arm raises [19–20] ▶
20. Kneeling Forward Bend (*Vajrāsana*) with head turns [55] ▶
39. Supine Abdominal Twist (*Jaṭhara Parivṛtti*) with leg adaptations [82] ▶

Eyes and Face

58. Eye stretches [113] <no video>
56. Lion (*Simhāsana*) [111] ▶

Breath Adaptations in Āsana

Metrical Inhale/Exhale Coordinated with Repetition of Movement

In the *Viniyoga* approach, repetitions of movement into and out of postures are often measured metrically using a predetermined length of count for inhale and exhale. This approach works beautifully for musicians in general and singers in particular because the regularity of breath and movement is so much like music. Moreover, attention to the count helps to keep attention in the moment and focused on the speed of breath and movement.

Use of Various Lengths of Inhale/Exhale

The traditional length of one count is one second; therefore, the speed of the count is metronome marking M.M. 60. Most posture repetitions work quite comfortably with a four-count inhale and four-count exhale. It is also useful to lengthen the count to six or eight, thereby slowing down the breath and movement and encouraging even more attention to the pace and smoothness of breath and movement. Breathing and moving at a slower pace also create more work, as the muscles must work smoothly rather than following the momentum of the movement. In addition, staying in a particular position at a longer breath count increases the effect of the posture.

It is also possible to speed up the count for a more vigorous workout or to make the count uneven for a particular purpose. For example, one could work on shortening the inhale and lengthening the exhale portion of the breath (necessary for singing long phrases) in order to practice taking full breaths quickly and then spinning out the breath over a much longer count. A one- or two-count inhale while raising the arms in *Tāḍāsana* followed by an eight-count exhale while lowering the arms would focus the attention completely on the long exhale and the smooth lowering of the arms. Here is an opportunity to see in the movement of the arms whether the exhale that will become tone in singing proceeds smoothly or has intermittent stops and starts or runs out before the end of the count.

Use of Krama (Segmenting the Breath)

Krama means to segment. The use of *krama* in breathing practices reveals exactly what parts of the major breathing muscles are working in a particular part of the breath (see chapter 3). The use of *krama* in *āsana* focuses attention closely on breath and movement and results in an improvement in muscular control. For example, using a four-count inhale and four-count exhale in *Tāḍāsana* (with arm and heel raises) with pauses between counts two and three effectively strengthens feet, legs, arms, and the breathing mechanism. Extending to three segments of a six-count inhale and exhale further slows down movement and gives more opportunities for muscular and breath control. Practices such as these also sharpen the focus of attention and provide a sense of being well grounded in the body.

Use of Ratio (Inhale/Suspend/Exhale/Suspend)

Ratio is the science of working with the breath in four parts: Inhalation (IN), Suspension with the lungs full (SF), Exhalation (EX), and Suspension with the lungs empty (SE). Inhalation is energizing, and suspension with the lungs full prolongs and intensifies this effect. Exhalation is calming, and suspension with the lungs empty prolongs and intensifies that effect. The concept of ratio is discussed more fully in chapter 3 and has many uses in breathing practices.

Ratio can also be used in *āsana* to intensify the effect of a particular posture. For example, using ratio in *Tāḍāsana* (with arm and heel raises) increases the energizing effects of the inhalation and provides a "stay" for building strength in the feet, legs, arms, and breathing mechanism. The calming effects of the exhalation are also increased, while the overall breath is lengthened considerably. When postures are practiced with a ratio, fewer repetitions are needed, as the ratio greatly intensifies the work being done.

Sample Sequences for Breath Adaptations in Āsana

♦ *A Sequence for Various Lengths of Metrical Breath Patterns*
▶ *Video demonstrations are of Warrior and Supine Forward Bend only*

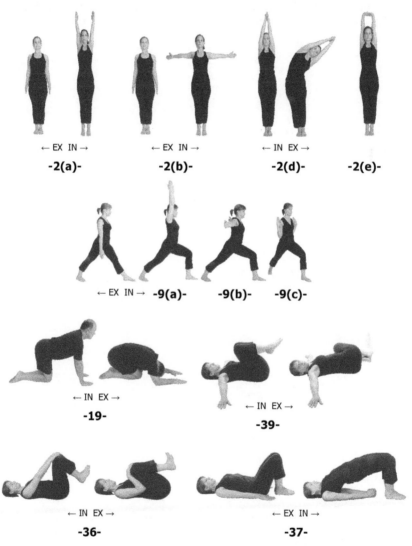

FIGURE 2.57 A Sequence for Various Lengths of Metrical Breath Patterns

2. Mountain with arm and heel raises: (a) x4, IN4/EX4; (b) x4, IN6/EX6; (d) x2 alternate sides, IN6/EX6; (e) stay 3 IN6/EX6 breaths

9. Warrior: (a) and (b) x2 each, IN3/EX6; (c) x2, IN6/EX6, stay 2 breaths

19. Ruddy Goose: x4; IN4/EX4, IN4/EX6, IN4/EX8, IN2/EX8

39. Supine Abdominal Twist: x4 each side; IN4/EX4, IN6/EX6, IN8/EX8 x2

36. Supine Forward Bend: x6; IN2/EX4, IN2/EX6, IN2/EX8 x2; IN1/EX8 x2

37. Bridge or Two-Footed Posture: x6; IN2/EX4, IN2/EX6, IN2/EX8 x2; IN1/EX8 x2

♦♦ *A Sequence for Krama* ⏵ *Video demonstrations are for Mountain (a) and Kneeling Forward Bend only*

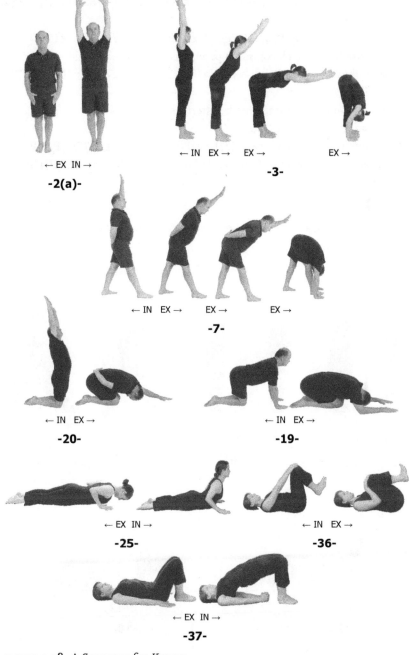

FIGURE 2.58 A Sequence for *Krama*

Breath pattern abbreviations: IN2/P/IN2/P (two segments) or EX2/P/EX2/P/
EX2/P (three segments) P = pause

2. Mountain with arm and heel raises: (a) x4; IN2/P/2/P/EX4 x2; IN6/EX2/
   P/2/P/2/P x2
3. Forward Bend: x4; IN4/EX2/P/2/P x2; IN6/EX2/P/2/P/2/P x2
7. Intense Side Stretch: x4; same pattern as 3. above; each side
20. Kneeling Forward Bend: x4; IN2/P/2/P; EX2/P/2/P x2; IN2/P/2/P/2/
    P; EX2/P/2/P/2/P x2
19. Ruddy Goose: x4; same breath pattern as 20.
25. Cobra: x2; IN2/P/2/P/EX4
36. Supine Forward Bend: x4; IN4/EX2/P/2/P x2; IN6/EX2/P/2/P/2/P x2
37. Bridge or Two-Footed Posture: x4; IN2/P/2/P/EX4 x2; IN2/P/2/P/2/P/
    EX6 x2

♦♦ *A Sequence for Ratio* ▶ *Video demonstration for Warrior (a) only*

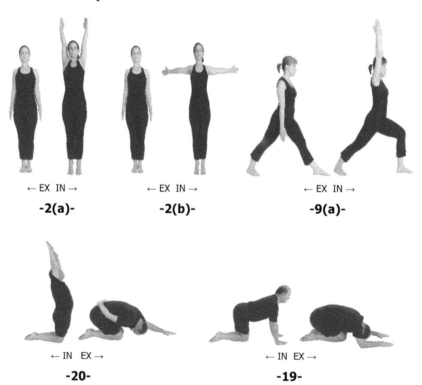

FIGURE 2.59 A Sequence for Ratio

Breathing ratio pattern (IN/SF/EX/SE) indicated with numbers only (4/2/4/2)

2. Mountain with arm and heel raises: (a) and (b) x4 each with 2:1:2:1 ratio: 4/2/4/2 x2; 6/3/6/3 x1; 8/4/8/4 x1
9. Warrior: (a) x4 with 2:1:4:1 ratio: 4/2/8/2 x2; 6/3/12/3 x1; 8/4/16/4 x1
20. Kneeling Forward Bend: x3 with 1:1:2:1 ratio: 2/2/4/2 x1; 4/4/8/4 x1; 6/6/12/6 x1
19. Ruddy Goose: x3 with 1:1:2:2 ratio: 2/2/4/4 x1; 3/3/6/6 x1; 4/4/8/8 x1

Sound in Asana

Traditionally, the use of sound in yoga practices consists mainly of chanting various Sanskrit texts. Chanting has several components: color of the sound, pitch, length, strength, consistency, and pattern. These elements can be varied to produce different energetic effects; that is, brighter color, higher pitch, shorter duration, fuller strength, and faster tempo will produce higher energy while darker color, lower pitch, longer duration, and slower tempo will have a calming effect. With respect to good health, the vibration set up by the use of the voice in chanting increases circulation in the body and contributes to the strength of the immune system.

There are various reasons to chant. Chanting helps to focus the mind, to set an intention, to train the attention, to train the voice, to learn something new, or to memorize something. All of these effects of chanting can be adapted to the needs of the singer on many levels. Moreover, using sounds and texts directly related to the elements of singing can easily replace Sanskrit texts.

Use of Vowel Sounds on Exhale in Repetition of Movement

Chanting in a seated position is the norm, but it is also possible to combine chanting with *āsana*. Using the repetition mode, the teacher intones a phrase while the class moves on inhalation, and the class repeats the phrase on the movement of exhalation. Adapting the practice of various postures with sound to the needs of the singer presents some interesting possibilities.

The most obvious adaptation is to use humming or spoken vowel sounds on the exhalation phase of the posture. This practice, if used with a varied length of inhale and a long exhale, will help to lengthen the breath span and the attention span needed for singing long phrases. The combination of movement with phonation makes learning more secure.

Another adaptation for the singer, especially for the American singer whose language uses diphthongs, is to use the movement of *āsana* to help focus the mind on saying or chanting absolutely pure vowels, especially [o] and [e] in which it is vital to keep the tongue, lips, and jaw in the same position for the duration of the sung vowel. Practicing these pure vowels in speech does not provide a long enough duration to duplicate singing the pure vowel throughout long tones, but practicing them in the context of slow movement replicates singing quite well. The physical movement itself reinforces the proper vowel sound.

French and German rounded front vowel sounds [y] [ʏ], [ø], [oe] can be practiced effectively in *āsana*. Unfamiliar consonant sounds, especially the German consonant sounds [ç] and [x] as well as many others, can also be practiced in this way. Practicing various unfamiliar sounds that occur in texts not in one's native language is an excellent way to supplement language diction classes, and can also help young singers who have not yet taken diction classes to learn the proper pronunciation of the songs they are singing.

Use as a Learning Device or to Sharpen Attention and Memory

The use of sound in *āsana* to learn something new can apply to learning new songs. To practice this approach, the yoga class could learn a song entirely new to the whole class in this call-and-response manner in the context of movement. In such a practice, mental attention will necessarily receive rigorous training.

The same approach can be taken to the process of memorization. Songs could be memorized one phrase at a time in one's individual *āsana* practice, using the repetitions of movement to repeat phrases or to string phrases together into sections or whole songs. Again, movement itself helps to solidify memory. In addition, the singer is practicing singing and moving at the same time, a skill necessary for the opera stage.

Sample Sequences for Sound in Āsana

A Sequence for Humming, Vowel, and Consonant Sounds

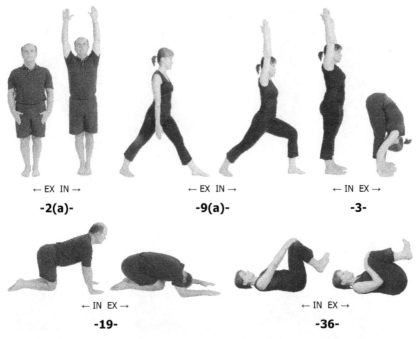

← EX IN →	← EX IN →	← IN EX →
-2(a)-	**-9(a)-**	**-3-**

← IN EX →	← IN EX →
-19-	**-36-**

FIGURE 2.60 A Sequence for Humming, Vowel, and Consonant Sounds

Use IN2/EX6 for all postures, listening on IN (or saying mentally if done in personal practice) and humming, saying vowel or consonant sounds on EX

2. Mountain with arm and heel raises: (a) x10: hum single tone x2; chant [a] x2; [ɛ] x2; [ɔ] x2; [u] x2
9. Warrior: (a) x6 each side; pure vowels: [e] x3; [o] x3
3. Forward Bend: x4; German "ch" sounds: [ç] x2; [x] x2
19. Ruddy Goose: x6; closed rounded front vowels: [y] x3; [ø] x3
36. Supine Forward Bend: x6; open rounded front vowels: [ʏ] x3; [oe] x3

A Sequence for Learning or Memorizing

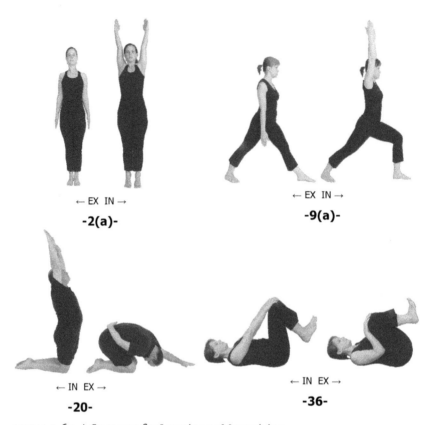

FIGURE 2.61 A Sequence for Learning or Memorizing

Choose any song or aria; use IN2/sing phrase; arrange order of phrases and repetitions to suit your needs; repeat phrases or string phrases together on repetitions.

2. Mountain with arm and heel raises: (a) x2–4; IN2/sing phrase 1
9. Warrior: (a) x2–4; IN2/sing phrase 2
20. Kneeling Forward Bend: x2–4; IN2/sing phrase 3
36. Supine Forward Bend: x2–4; IN2/sing phrase 4

3

Yoga and Singing

THE BREATH

Both rest on the foundation of awareness, control, and use of the breath.

Connections

In an article written in 1893, the famous Italian singing teacher G. B. Lamperti said, "The foundation of all vocal study lies in the control of the breath."[1] The great castrato Caffarelli is said to have spent six years on one page of vocalises prepared by his teacher Porpora to develop breath span, agility, and pure vowels.[2] Much of the voice student's time in lessons during the first year or two of study is spent on the issue of breath use—more if the student is not mindful of the breath in singing outside the studio. Breathing exercises apart from singing to develop the breathing mechanism tend to be unpopular with students, except for those very disciplined and dedicated to their own improvement.

The major issue in breath development for singers is the ability of the body and nervous system to tolerate highly irregular breath ratios with respect to inhalation and exhalation. Our normal autonomic breathing pattern is often referred to as the "tidal" breath—that is, the regular cycle of inhalation and exhalation. Under normal circumstances, the exhalation phase of the breath is slightly longer than the inhalation phase, and the relative lengths of each phase respond to the physical, mental, and emotional state of the moment. Under stress, the breath becomes shorter, higher in the chest, and somewhat restricted. Sometimes the breath is stopped or held in tense situations. In relaxed circumstances, the breath lengthens, deepens with relaxed abdominal muscles, and becomes looser. The singer must contradict almost all of these natural tendencies in order to practice the art of singing.

Foremost among the contradictions is that of learning to take a very short but full inhalation and then spin the breath out into tone over a much longer period of time. This requires physical and mental tolerance of the imbalance between lengths of inhalation and exhalation. This ability is developed in the creative practice of *prānāyāma* or yogic breathing practices. The second important contradiction that the singer must make is that of learning to relax under the stress of performing in order for the breath to work properly. This ability, too, is a learned skill that is fostered by various yoga practices.

We focus on how to take the breath but sometimes fail to follow through on how to use it in singing. Most often, breath use in a long phrase is related more to mindfulness of the vowel sound and will power than to how much breath has been taken. Students who lack mental focus will often suffer from short breath spans. Developing a long breath span is a specific goal of yogic breathing practices.

How to attend to the breath in the spaces between phrases is another area of concern. The ability to take long inhalations through the nose when time permits, or short, quick inhalations through the mouth where the music demands is a physical skill that can be developed apart from singing.

Refocusing on the breath at the end of each sung phrase is necessary for focused and consistent singing. The use of the breath as a focal point in concentration exercises develops this ability to return constantly to the breath in spite of all distractions. Total attention to *what* one is doing lessens the tendency to focus on *how* one is doing.

This use of the breath as a focal point in meditation practices reinforces the connection between a calm breath and a calm but alert mind—between calm breathing and an open heart. Awareness of the breath is also a component of deep relaxation exercises that open the whole person to a deep stillness in which all systems are renewed and from which all creative energy comes.

All these uses of the breath are addressed in specific yoga practices and, if practiced daily, become natural to the singer. Good health and the ease of daily life are also greatly enhanced (see table 3.1).

The Muscles of Breathing

The major muscles of breathing are

- the *diaphragm,* the dome-shaped muscle tissue separating the abdominal cavity from the thoracic cavity that arches up inside the ribs and connects to the lungs and the heart, as well as being attached to the lumbar vertebrae and to the lowest ribs
- the *rectus abdominus,* the long flat muscle (with four lateral divisions that give the "washboard" appearance) that originates at the pubic crest and

Table 3.1 Functions of the Breath

	In Life	In Yoga	In Singing
Physical:	Brings in oxygen to nourish every cell in the body and expels carbon dioxide.	Coordinates movement in and measures length of postures (*āsana*).	Stream of breath passing through the glottis sets up vibration of the vocal folds and produces sound; speed of the airflow determines ease of singing. Musically, each phrase demands a different length of breath; developing the ability to tolerate irregular breathing patterns is necessary.
Mental:	Affects the alertness of the brain and the functioning of the nervous system.	Use of breath as the focus of attention and awareness develops one-pointed concentration.	How the breath is used influences greatly the singer's state of mind and the functioning of the nervous system. Ability to refocus on the breath constantly is necessary.
Spiritual:	Breath is equated with both life and consciousness.	Focus on breath in meditation quiets the mind and opens the heart to the inner Self.	Artistically and expressively, a sense of total presence in singing depends on the ability to be fully present in the moment—a spiritual quality that can be nurtured using the tool of awareness of the breath.

inserts at the bottom of the sternum and the cartilage of the fifth, sixth, and seventh ribs

- the *internal* and *external obliques*, the abdominal muscles that lie diagonally on the sides of the trunk and are in opposition to each other, as well as working with the *rectus abdominus*
- the *internal* and *external intercostals*, the muscles between the ribs that elevate (opening the chest and creating more air space) and lower the ribs
- the *soft palate*, the muscular part of the roof of the mouth (lying behind the hard palate) that is movable for swallowing, speech, and respiration, among other uses; elevating the soft palate increases the space in the mouth for resonance.

Prānāyāma Practices for Breath Development and Control

There are numerous breathing practices (*prānāyāma*) that develop all the muscles of breathing as well as expansion and control of breath flow. In all the practices described below, the breath should be long and smooth. Any roughness or sudden instability of breath indicates stress. If this happens, either reduce the length of the breath or stop the practice. Never push the breath beyond its ability to remain calm and smooth.

Inhalation/Exhalation

The beginning point of the study and development of the breath for singing is the directional flow of Inhalation (IN) and Exhalation (EX). During *inhalation*, the directional flow of air is *downward;* during *exhalation*, the directional flow of air is *upward.* This is sometimes confusing to beginning singers because as the air flows in, the chest and abdominal muscles move out, and as air flows out, the abdominal muscles move in. An effective illustration of this principle is the examination of five different types of inhalation and three different types of exhalation, each of which focuses on muscular movement. In the following self-observation exercises, notice also the effect of different types of inhalation and exhalation on the movement of the spine, a crucial element in good singing posture. When the lower ribs are expanded, the spine extends and the chest opens; when the lower ribs collapse, the spine contracts and the chest sinks.

There is some disagreement about whether the spine extends or contracts during inhalation. Yogic sources refer to the extension of the spine during inhalation, whereas in a recent book on body mapping, *What Every Singer Needs to Know about the Body,* the author of the chapter on the singer's breath, Melissa Malde, states that the spine "gathers" or contracts on inhalation and lengthens on exhalation.³ In any case, the movement is subtle.

Five Types of Inhalation and Three Types of Exhalation

The following exercises should be practiced to a count of M.M. 60, the traditional speed of all the metrical patterns in yoga practices. In addition, many repetitions will establish M.M. 60 in the nervous system as a reference point for both yoga and musical practice.

Five types of inhalation

· Chest
· Belly
· Chest to belly (continuous flow)
· Belly to chest (continuous flow)
· Solar plexus, radiating out to chest and belly simultaneously

♦ **Self-observation exercise** ▶

· Sit in a comfortable position
· Place right hand on chest and left hand on belly
· With awareness in the chest, inhale 4 counts into the chest only and notice the right hand rising; repeat 4 times; notice effects in the spine
· With awareness in the belly, inhale 4 counts expanding the abdominal muscles only and notice the left hand rising; repeat 4 times; notice the effects in the spine and chest
· With awareness moving from chest to belly, inhale 2 counts into the chest, expanding the lower ribs, and 2 counts expanding the abdominal muscles; repeat 4 times; notice the effects in the spine
· With awareness moving from belly to chest, inhale 2 counts expanding the abdominal muscles and 2 counts into the chest, expanding the lower ribs; repeat 4 times; notice the effects in the spine
· With awareness at the solar plexus, inhale 4 counts into chest and belly simultaneously; repeat 4 times; notice the effects in the spine

Three types of exhalation

· Relaxed exhalation without abdominal contraction
· Exhalation with abdominal contraction

- Exhalation beginning with pulling up muscles of pelvic floor and contracting abdominals up to sternum

♦ **Self-observation exercise**
- Sitting comfortably, place right hand on chest and left hand on belly
- Inhale 4 counts and exhale 4 counts by simply relaxing the inhalation muscles; repeat 4 times; notice the effects in the spine
- Inhale 4 counts and exhale 4 counts by contracting the abdominal muscles, keeping the ribs expanded as long as possible; repeat 4 times; notice the effects in the spine
- Inhale 4 counts and exhale 4 counts by pulling up (contracting) the muscles of the pelvic floor and the abdominal muscles all the way up to the sternum; repeat 4 times; notice the effects in the chest and spine

The Singer's Breath

The "Singer's Breath" is usually a combination of chest and belly inhalation with the exhalation—the sung tone—being controlled by contracting the abdominal muscles while resisting the lowering of the ribs. Breathing high in the chest alone tends to limit air capacity and create tension in the throat, shoulders, and rib cage. Breathing low in the abdomen alone tends to pull the chest down. Breathing from the solar plexus and radiating upward to the ribs and downward to the belly may produce some unnecessary overall tension in the body. The remaining two ways to inhale—chest to belly, belly to chest— seem to be most favored by singers. Of the two, beginning the inhalation with rib expansion and finishing with belly expansion serves to open the chest immediately with the lifted lower ribs, providing extra space to take in more air with the abdominal expansion. Keeping the ribs expanded as long as possible without undue tension retains an open chest throughout the exhalation (sung) phase of the breath, allowing the abdominal muscles to contract inward and upward, keeping consistent breath pressure in the lungs to the end of the phrase. Therefore, it is this method of inhalation that is recommended for the breathing practices outlined later in the chapter.

Krama: Segmented Inhale and Exhale

As beginning singers are often unacquainted with the musculature involved in breathing for singing, especially the abdominal muscles, it is useful to practice *Krama*, or segmented breathing. *Krama* literally means "to segment." The concept can be applied to many different things in yoga practice—for example, to the repetition phase of many physical postures as a means of gaining greater muscular control of the body, as indicated in chapter 2.

The use of segmented breathing as a practice shows the singer precisely which parts of the abdominal muscles, especially the *rectus abdominus*, are working. Once these muscle parts are located, it becomes clearer what should be happening in the abdominal muscles during the sung phrase. Practicing *Krama* also strengthens the musculature with repetition.

It is interesting to note that Luisa Tetrazzini (1871–1940), the most famous coloratura soprano of her day and renowned for her breath control, practiced breathing in a segmented manner, which she described as follows: "Stand erect in a well-ventilated room or out of doors and slowly snuff in air through the nostrils, inhaling in little puffs, as if you were smelling something. Take just a little bit of air at a time and . . . when you have the sensation of being full up to the neck retain the air for a few seconds and then very slowly send it out in little puffs again."[4]

Krama: Segmented IN/EX—4 and 6 count ▶

♦ **A 4-count breath in 2 segments**

- Using a 4-count chest-to-belly IN, IN counts 1–2 expanding the lower ribs, pause, counts 3–4 expanding the abdominal muscles, pause
- Using a 4-count belly-to-chest EX *and keeping the ribs expanded throughout*, counts 1–2 contracting the belly muscles from pubis to navel, pause, counts 3–4 contracting from navel to sternum, pause
- Repeat 4 times

♦♦ **A 6-count breath in 3 segments**

- IN counts 1–2 expanding from sternum to solar plexus, pause, counts 3–4 expanding from solar plexus to navel, pause, counts 5–6 expanding from navel to pubis, pause
- EX, *keeping the ribs expanded throughout*, counts 1–2 contracting the abdominal muscles from pubis to navel, pause, counts 3–4 from navel to solar plexus, pause, counts 5–6 from solar plexus to sternum, pause
- Repeat 4 times

Breath Threshold

Breath threshold is one's maximum breath capacity (not the same as lung capacity) that changes according to inner and outer conditions; that is, one's maximum breath capacity will not be the same every day or even at different times on the same day. The average person breathes from fifteen to twenty times per minute. This rate can be changed, reduced up to 90 percent through conscious control of the respiratory system. Expanding the breath threshold is a necessity for singers because of the demands of long phrases. For example, a slow Mozart aria might demand only three breaths a minute, or even just two, depending on the tempo. The ability to sing long phrases comfortably can be developed with breathing practices designed to expand the breath threshold as well as to lengthen the exhalation phase of the breath. The following breath exploration and practice will allow the singer to find his or her personal threshold and then begin to expand it, reducing the number of breaths per minute.

♦ **Inhale and Exhale: Your personal maximum threshold**

· Sit comfortably with a straight spine, relaxed shoulders, head slightly back, chin slightly down
· Take 4 normal breaths
· Begin to deepen your IN and lengthen your EX to your comfortable maximum (e.g., IN8/EX8, or whatever is your personal maximum); take 4 breaths at your maximum, pausing 1 count between IN and EX
· Begin to shorten your IN and EX back to normal
· Note what your personal maximum breath length was
· The classic number of repetitions to determine whether the breath count you have chosen as your comfortable maximum is correct is twelve; if you cannot sustain your chosen breath length for twelve breaths without stress, practice a shorter breath length, working back up to your original length

♦ **A Short Practice to Expand the Breath Threshold**

· Keeping the spine straight, head a little back, chin a little down, shoulders relaxed, begin to deepen the IN and lengthen the EX in the pattern in chart 3.1, going only to your own limit (X = number of repetitions)

Chart 3.1

IN	EX	X	
4	4	4	Notice your comfortable capacity; at that
6	6	4	level, do 12 repetitions and then
8	8	4	return to normal breathing, working
10	10	4	backward through two repetitions each
12	12	4	of decreasing lengths of breath

Note: If at any time you feel light headed, dizzy, or nauseous during *prāṇāyāma*, stop immediately and resume normal breathing. Never push the breath. Go only to your comfortable limit for the day.

Ratio: Working with the Breath in Four Parts

Ratio is a mathematical pattern applied to breathing practices to lengthen the overall breath. These breathing patterns consist of four parts: Inhalation (IN), Suspension with the lungs full (SF), Exhalation (EX), and Suspension with the lungs empty (SE). (The *Viniyoga* designations for these four parts are Inhalation, Retention, Exhalation, Suspension; however, to avoid any sense of "holding" at the throat in the Retention phase, it is best for singers to think of Suspension of the breath with the lungs full. In fact, the *Yoga Sūtras* speak of these parts of the breath as Inhalation, Suspension with lungs full, Exhalation, and Suspension with lungs empty; thus, we are following an older tradition of nomenclature.) It is important to leave the glottis open during the suspension phases.

In yoga breathing practices there are certain effects of each of the four parts of the breath. Inhalation symbolically affects what lies above the diaphragm, and its effects are energizing, expanding, and vitalizing. Suspension of the breath after Inhalation prolongs and deepens the effects of Inhalation, including building strength in the muscles of inhalation. During Suspension after inhalation, the ribs are kept extended and the abdominal muscles out. The glottis is left open. Exhalation symbolically affects what lies below the diaphragm, and its effects are calming, grounding, and stabilizing. Suspension of the breath after Exhalation prolongs and deepens the effects of exhalation, also including building strength in the muscles of exhalation. Again, the glottis is left open in the suspension phase.

These effects of the four parts of the breath are of great importance to singers in building strength in the muscles of the breathing mechanism, in lengthening the overall breath, in lengthening the exhalation phase of the breath, and in building the mental focus and will power often needed to sustain a very long phrase. Using the tool of ratio, it is possible to strengthen, lengthen, and refine the control of the breath without the complications of singing at the same time.

The classic ratio in yoga breathing practice is 1:1:1:1, in which the four parts of the breath are equal. Ratio practices work up gradually to a goal length that is verified as being acceptable for the particular individual by repeating the goal breath twelve times. If it is not possible to repeat the breath twelve times without stress, the length of the breath is too long and should be reduced. (The classic goal is 10:10:10:10 repeated twelve times—a difficult achievement that should not be attempted without instruction in building up to this goal.) The following short ratio practice will introduce the concept at an easily achieved length. Sitting with a straight spine and relaxed body and counting at M.M. 60, follow the guide in chart 3.2 to work up to a sixteen-second breath, slightly less than four breaths per minute. Use the "chest to belly" inhalation, and keep the ribs expanded as long as possible on the abdominal exhalation.

A Short Ratio Practice @ 1:1:1:1 (1 = 4 sec.)

Chart 3.2

IN	SF	EX	SE	X
4	○	4	○	4
4	2	4	○	2
4	4	4	○	2
4	2	4	2	2
4	○	4	4	2
4	2	4	4	2
4	4	4	4	4–12
4	○	4	○	4

This short practice shows how ratio works. There are many other possible ratios for various purposes. In a 2:1:2:1 ratio, the Inhalation and Exhalation phases are equal, while the Suspension phases are half as long. In a 1:1:2:1 ratio, the Exhalation phase is lengthened, while the other three phases are equal. In a 1:1:2:2 ratio, the Exhalation phase is greatly lengthened by the addition of a longer Suspension with lungs empty. The ratio can be adjusted for a short Inhalation, say only one count for a full breath, a one-count suspension, a much longer exhalation, say sixteen counts, and a half-length suspension with the lungs empty. This ratio is similar to singing a long phrase on a full breath taken quickly at a short rest in the music. In all these and other ratios, one should begin with an easy length of count and increase it gradually, not going beyond the point at which it is possible to repeat the ratio twelve times without stress.

There are many possibilities of adaptation. For example, it is possible to design a breath ratio practice for a single troublesome phrase, such as the famous phrase, "Und die einsame Träne rinnt," in "Die Mainacht" by Johannes Brahms (see chart 3.3). The phrase is nineteen beats long—almost twenty seconds if Brahms's tempo marking of "Sehr langsam" is taken to be about M.M. 60. To assure success with the sung phrase, the goal length will be longer than twenty seconds, as actual tone demands more of the breath than voiceless breathing. The phrase is preceded by three beats of rest the first time it appears but only by an eighth rest the second time. The ratio will reflect this difference in the gradual shortening of the Inhalation/Suspension and lengthening of the Exhalation/Suspension parts of the ratio.

It is important to build up to the final ratio very gradually, as it is a strenuous practice. If the reader can already sing this phrase easily in one breath, it would be interesting to see what kind of experience this practice would be. It is also important to remember that other factors (such as efficiency of phonation, emotional involvement, dynamic level, and so forth) enter into singing such a phrase and that breath span alone, though it is foundational, may not be the complete solution to any problem with the phrase.

♦ ♦ ♦ Ratio Practice for "Und die einsame Träne rinnt"
(Brahms: "Die Mainacht")

Chart 3.3

IN	SF	EX	SE	X	
6	0	6	0	4	
6	3	6	3	4	Practice this part of the ratio until you are
6	4	6	4	4	able to do it comfortably before going on.
6	6	6	6	12	
Recovery Phase					
(see below)					
4	4	8	8	2	
4	4	10	10	2	Starting at the beginning (6-0-6-0) of the
3	3	12	12	4	ratio, work gradually up over a period of
2	2	12	10	2	days or weeks. Wherever you stop,
2	2	12	12	2	proceed to the recovery phase. Do not
1	1	12	10	2	simply return abruptly to normal
1	1	14	8	1	breathing.
1	1	16	6	1	
1	1	18	4	1	
1	1	20	2	4	
6	6	6	6	1	
6	4	6	4	1	Recovery Phase
6	3	6	3	1	
6	0	6	0	4	

Bandhas

Bandhas are muscular contractions (often called "locks") in specific parts of the body that function as strengthening agents, among other uses. There are three primary *Bandhas*: (1) *Jālandhara*, or chin lock, (2) *Uddīyāna*, or abdominal lock, and (3) *Mūla*, or root lock. *Bandhas* are an extension of *Prānāyāma* (breathing practices) and are usually taught after lengthening of the breath is well established. For singers, however, *Bandhas* are very useful for developing correct head posture and for greatly strengthening the muscles of exhalation and can be taught sooner.

The chin lock (*Jālandhara*) is applied *after inhalation* and consists of moving the head slightly back and the chin slightly down so that the head is in perfect alignment with the cervical spine and the back of the neck is lengthened. This is the proper head alignment for the most resonant singing. This lock in yoga practices may be stronger (chin lower) to develop the posture, but in actual singing the movement is whatever is needed for the individual singer to come into perfect alignment. Practiced on a regular basis for a few weeks, this *bandha* will make good head alignment much easier and more natural.

The abdominal lock (*Uddīyāna*) is applied *after exhalation* and consists of pulling all the abdominal muscles, from pubis to sternum, in and up as strongly as possible and keeping the contraction for a predetermined number of seconds. This action is done *when the lungs are empty, never when they are full*. This *bandha* is excellent for developing real strength in the abdominal muscles of exhalation that make it possible to sing long phrases comfortably. Practiced on a regular basis for a few weeks, it will develop strength quickly.

The root lock (*Mūla*) is usually applied after exhalation and consists of contracting the muscles of the pelvic floor (those between the anus and the genitals) upward toward the navel. It is an agent for strengthening the pelvic floor muscles as well as the lower abdominal muscles. This lock is especially useful to singers in a subtle way. When applied immediately after inhalation and before beginning the sung phrase, the support of the root lock enhances the clarity of the tone and gives firmness to the subsequent support of the phrase. It is more difficult than one imagines to keep the root lock in position for more than a few seconds, especially while doing something else—like singing. Therefore, practicing this lock on a regular basis will develop the ability to sustain it for longer periods of time.

Before *Bandhas* can be practiced successfully in the context of *prānāyāma*, it is necessary to be able to sustain an 8-count (ideally a 10-count) breath in a 1:1:1:1 ratio for four repetitions; that is, eight counts each of Inhalation, Suspension with lungs full, Exhalation, and Suspension with lungs empty.

This gives sufficient time to apply each lock and keep it long enough to build muscular strength. A short *bandha* practice will illustrate the technique (see chart 3.4).

Note: There are some contraindications applicable to practicing *bandhas*. Anyone with severe digestive tract disease should be cautious about practicing *Uddīyāna Bandha* as well as women who are pregnant.

♦ ♦ ♦ *Bandhas*: A short practice

Chart 3.4

IN	SF	EX	SE	X	
4	1*	4	1	4	* lower chin and pull head back slightly
4+	2	4	2	4	+ keep chin lock throughout remainder of
6	3	6	3	4	practice
8	4	8	4∧	4	∧ engage abdominal lock and release
8	8	8	8∧∧	4	before next IN
8	o	8	o	1	∧∧ engage root and abdominal locks
6	o	6	o	1	and release before next IN

Techniques: The Use of Different "Valves"

A breathing technique in yoga is the use of a valve to regulate the flow of breath. Valves are openings through which a liquid or gas passes in one direction at a time. The two main valves through which air passes in the breathing process are the throat and the nostrils. A third valve used in yoga breathing practices is the curled tongue for inhalation. These three valves, separately or in combination, are used in specific ways for specific effects.

It is useful to realize that the throat valve, at the proper closure, produces phonation when breath passes out through it. A very slight firming of the vocal folds during inhalation or exhalation produces a light sound of rushing air. The use of this "sound breath" is called *Ujjāyī*, and is used quite often in physical postures as well as in various breathing techniques. In actuality, the air inhaled and exhaled with *Ujjāyī* comes through both nostrils, as the mouth remains closed, though it is often referred to as breathing through the throat.

The use of this slight sound serves both to regulate the flow of breath and as a focus for attention. The sound can be loud, soft, or inaudible, depending on the reason for its use. Its effect is that of producing heat. Singers should use a moderate level of *Ujjāyī*, but not immediately before a performance, as it can be drying to the vocal folds.

The nostrils as valves have many uses in breathing practices. They can be used together or separately, with the proper hand technique for closing and opening each nostril. The use of alternate nostrils is accomplished by manipulating the opening and closing with the thumb and ring finger of the right hand. The most common form of the hand use is to fold down the first two fingers of the right hand and place them on the tip of the nose. The thumb then manipulates the right nostril, and the ring and little fingers manipulate the left nostril. This is an easy way to open and close the nostrils alternately. Another form of this technique is to place the first two fingers of the hand on the forehead at the bridge of the nose and use the thumb and ring finger to manipulate the nostrils. Either way works well. The main reason either to fold the first two fingers down or place them on the forehead is to get them out of the way.

For the student unacquainted with breathing practices in general, it is advisable to begin with a qualified teacher, as incorrect or excessive use of breathing practices can have an undesirable effect on the nervous system. Contraindications for alternate nostril practices include blocked nostrils or sinuses (although gentle practice will often open slightly blocked nasal passages), congestion in the lungs, upper respiratory or other illness, headache, extreme fatigue, or after eating a meal.

Four Alternate Nostril Breathing Practices

There are four primary practices that use alternate nostrils as valves. Three use the nostrils in alternation with the throat, and one uses alternate nostrils only. Each practice has a specific effect on the nervous system and can be used in many different situations.

Anuloma Ujjāyī is a breathing technique that uses the throat sound (*Ujjāyī*) for inhalation and alternate nostrils for exhalation. The word *anuloma* means "with the hair," referring to the direction in which the hairs inside the nostrils grow. The movement of air during exhalation is in the direction of hair growth, and the effect of this breath on the nervous system is calming. The hand may be raised to close the appropriate nostril in exhalation and lowered for inhalation. A short *Anuloma Ujjāyī* practice illustrates the technique (see chart 3.5).

♦ *Anuloma Ujjāyī:* A Short Practice (Inhale throat, exhale
alternate nostrils) ▶

Chart 3.5

IN *U*	EX *l*	IN *U*	EX *r*	X
4	4	4	4	4
6	6	6	6	4
8	8	8	8	4–12
6	6	6	6	4
4	4	4	4	4

U (Ujjāyī) = throat; *l* = left nostril; *r* = right nostril

Viloma Ujjāyī is a breathing technique that uses alternate nostrils for inhalation and the throat for exhalation. The word *viloma* means "against the hair,"
referring to the movement of air during inhalation in the opposite direction of
hair growth, and the effect of this breath on the nervous system is energizing.
The hand may be raised to close the appropriate nostril for inhalation and
lowered for exhalation. A short *Viloma Ujjāyī* practice illustrates the technique
(see chart 3.6).

♦ *Viloma Ujjāyī:* A Short Practice (Inhaling alternate nostrils, exhaling
throat) ▶

Chart 3.6

IN *l*	EX *U*	IN *r*	EX *U*	X
4	4	4	4	4
6	6	6	6	4
8	8	8	8	4–12
6	6	6	6	4
4	4	4	4	4

U (Ujjāyī) = throat; *l* = left nostril; *r* = right nostril

In case the explanation of the terms *anuloma* and *viloma* above seem far-
fetched, consider the action of stroking a cat's fur. Stroking in the direction of
hair growth is pleasing and calming to the cat; stroking against the direction

of hair growth is irritating to the cat and will often produce energetic effects. The same can be said of stroking versus touseling the hair of a person.

Nāḍī Śodhana is a breathing technique that uses the nostrils alternately for both inhalation and exhalation. The hand is kept at the nostrils for the entire practice. A round of *Nāḍī Śodhana* consists of inhaling through the left nostril, exhaling through the right nostril, inhaling through the right, and exhaling through the left. Suspensions may be inserted after inhalations and exhalations. This technique works well with a ratio. The effect of this breath on the nervous system is balancing. A short *Nāḍī Śodhana* practice illustrates the technique (see chart 3.7).

♦♦ *Nāḍī Śodhana*: A Short Practice with Ratio ▶

Chart 3.7

IN *l*	SF	EX *r*	SE	IN *r*	SF	EX *l*	SE	X
4	1	4	1	4	1	4	1	1
4	2	4	2	4	2	4	2	1
4	4	4	4	4	4	4	4	2
6	3	6	3	6	3	6	3	1
6	4	6	4	6	4	6	4	1
6	6	6	6	6	6	6	6	2–6*
8	4	8	4	8	4	8	4	1
8	6	8	6	8	6	8	6	1
8	8	8	8	8	8	8	8	2–6
8	0	8	0	8	0	8	0	2
6	0	6	0	6	0	6	0	2

[*r* = right nostril; *l* = left nostril]

* 6 if stopping here; 2 if continuing

Pratiloma Ujjāyī is a more complex breathing technique that uses inhalation and exhalation through both throat and alternate nostrils in a pattern that is completed on the left side before repeating it on the right side. This practice is a combination of the qualities of calming and energizing and may have different effects on different people. A short *Pratiloma Ujjāyī* practice will serve as an introduction to its effects (see chart 3.8).

♦ ♦ ♦ *Pratiloma Ujjāyī* : A Short Practice—Building the Exhale and Refining Attention

Chart 3.8

IN *U*	EX *l*	IN *l*	EX *U*	IN *U*	EX *r*	IN *r*	EX *U*	X
4	4	4	4	4	4	4	4	2
4	6	4	6	4	6	4	6	2
4	8	4	8	4	8	4	8	2
6	6	6	6	6	6	6	6	2
6	10	6	10	6	10	6	10	1
6	12	6	12	6	12	6	12	1
6	6	6	6	6	6	6	6	1
4	4	4	4	4	4	4	4	2

(*l* = left nostril; *r* = right nostril; *U* = throat; no suspensions)

Śītalī is a breathing practice in which air is inhaled through the extended curled tongue and exhaled through alternate or both nostrils with the tip of the tongue curled upward to touch the palate. The effect on the nervous system is cooling. This technique is also useful in exercising the muscles of the soft palate, as the soft palate must remain raised throughout the exhalation. A short *Śītalī* practice will illustrate the technique (see chart 3.9).

♦ ♦ *Śītalī:* A Short Practice ▶

· Lower the chin and extend the tongue, curling the sides to make a straw-like tunnel
· Inhale through the curled tongue (air will be cool) while raising the chin slightly above level
· Curl the tongue back upon itself until the bottom of the tip is touching the palate; lower the chin
· Close the right nostril with the hand and exhale through the left
· Repeat inhalation through curled tongue
· Fold tongue back and exhale through the right nostril

Chart 3.9

IN *ct*	EX *l*	IN *ct*	EX *r*	X
4	4	4	4	4

ct = curled tongue

Other Breath-Related Practices

Just as *bandhas* are intimately connected with the breath, though they themselves are not breathing practices, so there are some cleansing techniques that make use of the breath, one of which is *Kapālabhāti* (♦ ♦). This practice is said to clear the nasal passages and to energize a sluggish mind. It is sometimes called the "Skull Shining" breath. This cleansing technique consists of a normal inhalation through both nostrils followed by a forceful exhalation (powered by a quick inward pull of the abdominal muscles), also through both nostrils. Several rounds of this technique should be followed by several slow, deep breaths to avoid excessive pressure through the nose and any tendency to become dizzy. It is a useful practice to clear the mind as well as the nostrils.

Humming

The yogic breathing practice called the "Bee Breath" (*Bhrāmarī*) uses a light humming sound (like that of the black bee) on the exhalation and is said to produce "a most harmonious voice."[5] This breathing practice is the first connector of the breathing practices to actual phonation and thus to singing. Humming is an extension of *prānāyāma* that uses sound to control the length of exhalation. It engages the intrinsic muscles of the larynx in a light and smooth way (if done *pianissimo* and felt at the bridge of the nose rather than loudly and felt in the throat) and is a beneficial vocal exercise for many purposes.

The use of the properly placed *pianississimo* hum is recognized by many voice therapists as a remedy for excessive sub-glottal pressure and other physiological problems in singing or speaking. A *pianississimo* hum activates only the two outer layers of the vocal folds (where most vocal pathologies occur). Moreover, Jean Westerman Gregg, voice teacher and speech-language pathologist who wrote the column "From Song to Speech" for the National Association of Teachers of Singing *Journal of Singing* for many years, makes a strong case for humming as a part of the voice building process as well as a therapeutic tool.[6] Enrico Caruso, in the book *Caruso and Tetrazzini on The Art of Singing*, first published in 1909, strongly recommended singing "with the mouth shut" as a method of properly placing the voice, gaining breath control and agility, restoring a damaged voice, and saving the voice itself for performance demands.[7] Also fostered by humming are relaxed jaw, tongue, and shoulders. Humming is an excellent way to warm up the voice and to practice certain passages in actual music, provided the hum is effortlessly placed. One should hum only as high as comfortable without facial, neck, or tongue tension.

In addition, a study by Eddie Weitzberg, an associate professor at the Karolinska Institute in Stockholm, and his colleagues showed that humming increases airflow within the sinuses. This increases the level of nitric oxide gas within the nose. "We believe that nitric oxide might help keep the sinuses clean from bacteria, since higher concentrations of this gas can kill bacteria."[8] Including humming in daily yoga practice seems to be healthful for the voice in numerous ways.

Patterns and Songs

Humming various vocalise patterns not only warms up the voice and helps to find a high resonance focus but also extends the breath span, encourages a smooth and supple singing line, and trains accuracy in pitch. The following basic humming exercises can be elaborated upon according to the singer's own needs and creative imagination. The use of humming "My Country, 'Tis of Thee" (*America*) or a comparable well-known song as far as possible on one breath establishes a benchmark for the singer's present breath span. After several weeks or months of *prāṇāyāma* practice, including humming, the benchmark should become an easy achievement. At this point, the singer should try a longer song with larger intervals, such as "America, the Beautiful" (*Materna*), on one breath. The possibilities are endless. From humming exercises, it is a natural transition to the use of full sound in *āsana* sequences.

Humming Exercises ▶

- ◆ Humming long tones: begin on a comfortable tone and hum 4, 6, 8, 12, 16 counts; move up or down by half-step until your comfortable limits are reached 🔲 ▶
- ◆ Humming arpeggios: begin on your lowest tone and hum 1-3-5-8-5-3-1; 1-4-6-8-6-4-1; 1-5- b7-8- b7-5-1; experiment with 1, 2, or 4 counts per pitch, and hum the entire arpeggio on one breath; repeat, going up by half-steps until you have reached your upper limit 🔲 ▶
- ◆ ◆ Humming wide intervals: begin on your lowest comfortable chest voice tone and hum 1-8-1-10-1-12-1-16-12-10-8-5-3-1, going up by half steps until you reach your comfortable upper limit (this exercise will take you through all of your vocal registers); experiment with 1 and 2 counts per pitch, and hum the entire exercise on one breath 🔲 ▶
- ◆ Humming major scale intervals: 1-2-1-3-1-P4-1-P5-1-6-1-7-1-8-1; 8-7-8-6-8-5-8-4-8-3-8-2-8-1 (repeat throughout your range); at 1 or 2 counts per pitch, hum the ascending form on one breath, then the descending form on one breath 🔲 ▶
- ◆ ◆ Humming minor scale intervals: 1-2-1-b3-1-4-1-5-1-b6-1-b7-1-8-1; 8-b7-8-b6-8-5-8-4-8-b3-8-2-8-1; at 1 or 2 counts per pitch, hum the

ascending form on one breath and the descending form on one breath 🔲 ▶

- • ◆ ◆ ◆Humming chromatic intervals: ascending: 1-m2-1-M2-1-m3-1-M3-1P4-1-Aug.4-1-P5-1-m6-1-M6-1-m7-1-M7-1-8; descending: 8-m2-8-M2-8-m3-8-M3-8-P4-8-Aug.4-8-P5-8-m6-8-M6-8-m7-8-M7-8-1; at 1 count per pitch, hum the ascending form on one breath and the descending form on one breath 🔲 ▶
- • ◆Humming scales: (on one breath at various counts per pitch)
- • Major scale: 1-2-3-4-5-6-7-8-7-6-5-4-3-2-1 🔲 ▶
- • Natural Minor scale: 1-2-b3-4-5-b6-b7-8-b7-b6-5-4-b3-2-1 🔲 ▶
- • Harmonic Minor scale: 1-2-b3-4-5-b6-7-8-7-b6-5-4-b3-2-1 🔲 ▶
- • Melodic Minor scale: 1-2-b3-4-5-6-7-8-b7-b6-5-4-b3-2-1 🔲 ▶
- • ◆"My Country, 'Tis of Thee" on one breath (use as a benchmark for initial breath span and a yardstick for progress in lengthening the breath)
- • ◆ ◆"America the Beautiful" on one breath
- • ◆ ◆ ◆"The Star-Spangled Banner" on two breaths
- • Any vocalizing patterns may be used with humming
- • Troublesome phrases of songs may be hummed to discover the exact location of the problem, whether it is breath, tonal focus, pitch, or register.

The Breath as a Focal Point

The breath is the most immediate point of life. In fact, breath is life, for without it we have no earthly existence. It is also the primary connector between body and mind and, as such, is used as a focal point in many yoga practices that deal with developing the mind into a one-pointed instrument for living. The breath is used as a focal point in physical postures, breathing practices, concentration exercises, meditation, and deep relaxation techniques. In most of these elements, the primary activity is repeatedly returning the attention and awareness to the breath as many times as the mind is distracted by its own activity.

This mental practice of returning the focus repeatedly to the breath is invaluable as a tool for training singers in the ability to refocus constantly on the work of the breath in singing. All too often, unseasoned singers become distracted by inner thoughts or outer events and forget the breath during performance. The smooth flow of breath and tone go hand in hand with the smooth flow of awareness, and disruption of the latter usually results in disruption of the former. Therefore, it is of great importance for the singer to train the mind in awareness, focus, and presence with the tool of the breath.

4

Yoga and Singing

THE MIND

Both demand mental concentration and the ability to coordinate mind and body.

Yoga is the control of thought waves in the mind.[1]

Connections

As a voice teacher, I cannot count the times I have stopped a student in a lesson, patiently re-explained something for the umpteenth time, and asked the student to repeat the vocalise (often a phenomenon of vocalizing when many singers take the opportunity to think of something else!). The repetition is flawless. In answer to my question, "What were you doing differently?" the student says, "Thinking," or "Oh, I was just focusing." Depending on the level of my frustration, I would reply, "Imagine that!" or "What a concept!" or something more colorful. This is a concrete example of the principle of acting with *mindfulness* as opposed to mindlessness.

The body is our vehicle for living, the physical form in which we move and do our work and enjoy the world. The mind is our instrument for living, the mental director and coordinator of all the body does. The mind directs the show and has many different modes and functions. We have a thinking mode in which we think through, plan, coordinate, and execute activities. We have a focus of attention mode in which we focus on the task at hand, whatever it may be. We also have an awareness mode in which we are aware of the present moment to the exclusion of past or future moments.

This awareness mode often needs special training because we are educated to be mentally active, analytical, and rational most of the time. The awareness mode seems to be more natural to creative artists of all kinds, perhaps because their creations so often come through this mode of the moment-to-moment awareness of being. This ability to be "in the moment" is a hallmark of all truly great performers, the quality that makes the transmission of their art seem to be for each individual receiver only. We call this quality "presence." It is a spiritual quality that can be developed in concentration practices and nourished in meditation. Yoga offers many different concentration techniques that train the mind to be "one-pointed," that give the person mastery over the mind rather than letting the ever-active and distracting mind have mastery over the person.

The Mind of a Singer

If the brain of an operatic singer onstage during performance could be mapped with electrodes, it is probable that almost every area would light up in bright colors. Chapter 1 gives a partial description of the facets of the person that the operatic singer must use—all at the same time—during performance. There is hardly any system that is not "on"—a superb example of multitasking, yet one that must be completely focused in the moment as if it were a single thing. It is little wonder that training for this profession takes many years.

It has been said that the three requirements for an operatic career are voice, voice, and voice. That, of course, is the first requirement and may have sufficed in the first three and a half centuries or so of the operatic art form. From the advent of the first televised opera, however, and increasingly in our visual age, the voice must be matched by a mind trained to coordinate many artistic abilities into the art of aurally and visually convincing performance at the close range of the television camera as well as on stage.

Even the most gifted require training, and many fail for lack of discipline. It is a common observation that the most disciplined singers sometimes lack the spontaneous freedom and openness to communicate well in performance, while the open and spontaneous personalities sometimes lack the discipline to perfect the instrument for their desire to communicate. So it is that the great coordinator of all singing activities, the mind, must be trained for both disciplined focus and open awareness.

The Coordinator

As the instrument of coordination, the mind must first develop a friendly and observant connection with the body. Many singers seem not to have good body awareness, especially if they have never played any sport successfully. Yoga's physical postures (*āsanas*) attune the mind to the parts of the body being worked in each posture while strengthening or freeing that particular part. Focusing nonjudgmentally on the effects of the posture develops a healthy respect for the body that promotes both acceptance and good health. As the postures become more comfortable and natural, mental focus can open to an overall awareness of stability and ease, the two traditional goals in *āsana* practice. This feeling of stability and ease will, over time, begin to transfer to other activities, including singing.

The Instrument of Learning

As the instrument of learning, the mind of the singer has many tasks. In addition to learning the elements of good vocal technique and embedding them in the body and nervous system, the mind must take on the task of learning music—pitches and rhythms, words and meanings, foreign languages and perhaps different ways of pronouncing one's own language. Then comes the task of memorizing, using yet another ability of the mind—accurate storage of the information learned. All of these tasks require a well-focused mind. It is commonly accepted that a short period of mentally focused work will yield more and better results than a longer period of distracted half-work. If the singer's mind is not finely focused in study and practice, much time will be wasted, and the habit of mindless singing is more likely to carry over into performance. The need is the ability to ignore distractions arising from within or entering through the senses.

The One-Pointed Mind

In yoga, the most common description of a well-functioning mind is "one-pointed." In other words, the fully trained mind can be used very selectively to focus, like a laser beam, on a single point without distraction. Some people seem able to do this naturally, but for most of us, training is needed at some point in our lives. Yoga practices are replete with techniques for developing a one-pointed focus that allows undistracted attention in the moment.

Performance anxiety in its various forms finds easy entry to a scattered or distracted mind. A scattered mind is one that tends to be aware of many things at the same time and has difficulty focusing on just one of them. A distracted mind may attend either to inner distractions (old memories, present discomforts or fears, future dreams) or outer distractions (what is happening at the moment in one's immediate environment).

A mind untrained in one-pointedness will be easily sidetracked from the business at hand. Those neutral or even positive thoughts that distract the mind merely hinder the performer. Negative thoughts and feelings that usually have their roots in the past can be destructive and sometimes debilitating to the performer. The key is to train the mind to ignore distractions and stay in the present moment.

The Relaxed Mind

It may seem contradictory to speak of the mind's being both one-pointed and relaxed at the same time, but the two states are complementary and bring the person to a state of balanced readiness—a state of equilibrium that feels like total freedom. It is common to hear Olympic athletes refer to their worst performances as results of being tense and tight and their best performances as results of being relaxed. Obviously, the moments before performance are focused, but that focus can be tense and fearful or relaxed and free. The relaxation begins in the mind and flows into the nervous system, freeing the body to respond at the highest levels of ability. The singer's performance is no different from the athlete's in this respect.

The concentration techniques of yoga are preliminary to meditation and culminate in deep relaxation in which all systems of the body and mind are rested and renewed. Entering this state of relaxed awareness on a regular basis will, in time, carry over into daily activities, including singing.

The Mind Trained for Performance

It is clear that the mind of the singer must be trained in many different ways. It must coordinate the body in the act of singing as well as in movement. It must learn music, words, unfamiliar pronunciations, meanings, characters, staging, and the sequence of events in a performance. It must coordinate its own work with that of others in ensemble situations and respond to unexpected events. It must be able to focus on a single thing while remaining aware of many other things. It must be able to let go of the past, put aside present distraction, and remain in the moment. It must be in a relaxed state to allow all these things to happen in a smooth and continuous flow. The daily practice of all the elements of classical yoga provides the training for these needs. In addition, such practice benefits the whole person in all of life's facets and makes living easier and more joyful.

Concentration Practices

The practices in this section focus on training the mind to let go of uninvited or unwanted thoughts, feelings, memories, or undesirable habits and also on the process of forming new habits. The practice for setting a new direction creates the mental environment for taking stock of one's life up to the present time and then looking forward in time to imagine the future.

◆ *For Mental Focus*

- A practice of noticing and letting go of unwanted thoughts and feelings—the initial step in learning to control the "thought waves" in the mind
- Choose an object for your mental focus—anything that interests you:
  - a physical object: for example, a rose; as you focus on the rose, notice all its physical characteristics, and allow all the associations you have with the rose to come to mind, including traditional meanings of the rose; allow your mind to become completely absorbed in the rose
  - a word: something that has meaning for you; as you focus on the word, allow all the associations you have with the word to come to mind; become completely absorbed in the word
  - a sound: for example, wind in leaves or water flowing over rocks, or a musical tone; as you focus on the sound, allow your mind to become completely absorbed in the sound
  - the breath: for example, the sensation of the breath flowing in the nostrils; as you focus on the breath, notice when it is cool and when it is warm, the beginning, middle, and end of each inhalation and each exhalation, and the space in between; become completely absorbed in the sensations of breathing
- Sitting with straight spine, head a little back and chin a little down, relaxed forehead muscles, jaw, tongue, shoulders and arms, eyes closed, establish a smooth flowing 6-count IN/6-count EX
- Focus mentally on the chosen object, keeping your breath long and smooth
- When thoughts or feelings arise and your attention wanders, notice where your attention went, and return your awareness to the object of focus
- Continue this oscillation from distraction to focus for several minutes

◆ ◆ *For Weakening and Letting Go of Old Thought Habits*[2]

- Attention on the old disturbance or stressful situation associated with the old thought habit
- Objectless attention
- Alternation between the two
- Sitting with straight spine, relaxed forehead muscles, jaw, tongue, shoulders and arms, closed eyes, lengthen the breath to IN6/EX6

- Focusing on the breath at the nostrils, take six breaths without losing your focus
- Now allow your mind to rest without judgment or emotion on the old habit you have chosen; when your mind wanders, move your focus back to the breath or simply to no focus at all
- When your mind wanders from the breath or from no focus, return your focus to the old habit
- Repeat this oscillation back and forth for a few moments
- End with resting your focus on the breath

♦♦ For Forming New Habits[3]

- Objectless attention
- Attention on the desired new habit
- Alternation between the two
- Sitting with straight spine, relaxed forehead muscles, jaw, tongue, shoulders and arms, closed eyes, lengthen the breath to IN6/EX6
- Focusing on the breath at the nostrils, take six breaths without losing your focus
- Now allow your mind to rest on the breath or on no focus at all; when your mind wanders, move your focus to the new habit you want to form
- When your mind wanders from the focus, return to the breath or to no focus at all
- Repeat this oscillation back and forth for a few moments
- End with resting your focus on the desired new habit

♦♦♦ For Setting a New Direction[4]

- Image of the flowing river
- Look backward to beginning of journey
- Look at the present
- Look downstream to desired goal
- Sitting with straight spine, relaxed forehead muscles, jaw, tongue, shoulders and arms, closed eyes, lengthen the breath to IN6/EX6
- Focusing on the breath at the nostrils, take six breaths without losing your focus
- Allow the image of a flowing river to come to mind
  - Begin to imagine your life as this flowing river
  - Look back upstream to the source of your life at birth; note all the people, family and friends, who were important in your early life Mark your first introduction to the direction you are now taking

- Remember your experiences and the feelings you have had up to now about this direction
- Remember all the teachers and friends who have helped you on your way
- *Do 6 more rounds of IN6/EX6*
- As the view of your life flows on, look at where you are right now. How have all your choices led you to this moment? How have they affected your direction?
- *Do 6 more rounds of IN6/EX6*
- Now look downstream as the river of your life flows into the future. Where do you want to go? Will your present direction take you there? How will your choices today affect tomorrow? Can you continue on your present course, or should you set a new course?
- *Do 6 more rounds of IN6/EX6;* then allow the mind to rest in simple awareness

5

Yoga and Singing

THE HEART

Both open the heart.

Connections

Singing is an overflow of the spirit—a matter of the heart. It is something "transmitted as an offering" from the singer to the listener. If the heart is fearful or closed, the transmission of the offering will be far less than it can be. The meditation practices of yoga address not only stillness of mind but also openness of heart and the self-knowledge and deep joy that is found there.

The Heart of the Singer

Every singer has some profound need to sing, and most have a strong desire to communicate what they feel to others. The heart plays perhaps the most vital role in all great singing, for if the singing does not come from the heart, it seems detached or even cold to the listener, merely an exercise in beautiful sound. Some singers have the need and the desire but are afraid to open the heart in a way that is self-revealing. These are the singers who need practices that open the heart and lead to self-acceptance and a sense of empowerment. Other singers are too emotional to open the heart for fear of losing control. These also need practices that open the heart and allow the singer to be with the emotion until it is resolved and can be transmuted into the emotional gold of expressive performance.

The heart plays a major role in understanding the meaning in poetry. Beyond the understanding of words and their definitions, a function of the mind, there is something that says "yes" to the truth of a poem. We commonly think of this as the heart's recognition. Song texts are not always easy to grasp, though well-composed music of a composer who understands the poetry usually leads the way and expresses specific elements of the text. In order to understand, we think of such things as learning the text "by heart," of living with the text, of relating it to our own experiences, of letting it sink into the understanding of the heart. We also think of learning music "by heart," and since music by itself does not engage words, we understand and feel the music at the heart level.

Once the singer advances beyond student literature, he or she will encounter songs and texts and operas that go beyond already experienced musical and poetic territory—indeed, beyond personal life experience. This requires the singer to be open to many new thoughts and experiences. In the process of entering new territory, the singer will almost certainly find much uncharted and sometimes unsettling territory within himself or herself. This requires openness to the new and different and a fearlessness that allows entry to these realms. Fearlessness is a quality that is needed by every performer in many different situations. It is a quality that can be cultivated with sufficient meditation practice.

These needs of the heart—communicating emotion, understanding, openness, and fearlessness—are all addressed in one way or another in the practice of meditation, which is the goal of all the other yoga practices. *Āsana* prepares for *prāṇāyāma*, *prāṇāyāma* prepares for concentration, and concentration prepares for meditation.

Meditation

All true artists, whether they know it or not, create from a place of no-mind, from inner stillness.[1]

Meditation is the practice of entering into inner stillness and silence. It follows naturally the process of one-pointed concentration sustained over a sufficient period of time that the mind becomes quiet and thoughts cease for brief moments. It is during these brief moments of inner silence that the work of untying mental or emotional knots begins to happen. These knots are the conditioned habits of our lives that do not serve us well, or that actually block our progress in development of all kinds. In his book *Yoga for Transformation*, Gary Kraftsow addresses this facet of meditation practice: "As we can influence our physical structures through the intelligent practice of *āsana* and our energy through the intelligent practice of *āsana* and *prāṇāyāma*, so too we can influence our personality through the practice of meditation."[2]

Performance anxiety is a case in point. Except for that which comes from being unprepared, most serious performance anxiety is rooted in the past and consists of mental and emotional knots that stand squarely between the singer and the singing. Once the particular knots have been identified, it is possible to begin the work of untying them in the practice of meditation.

At the Waisman Laboratory for Brain Imaging and Behavior in Madison, Wisconsin, ongoing experiments in mapping the brains of experienced meditators are beginning to show scientific evidence of the way meditation works to change habits by weakening the synapses in the brain associated with those habits. A major participant in the Wisconsin study was a young Tibetan monk, Yongey Mingyur Rinpoche, trained from the age of five in traditional Tibetan meditation practices and tutored by the scientists among his father's Western students in cutting edge Western scientific knowledge. His book, *The Joy of Living*, is a fascinating look into the intersection of ancient practices and modern science. For the Western mind that insists on knowing the "how" of the results of mental practices, this book is a valuable resource.

A main point of consistent meditation practice is that the accumulation of the mental effects of even the briefest periods of stillness and silence begin, over time, to change the way one perceives daily events and thus how one responds to them. Most often the first clue that change is happening is that the habitual reaction to certain triggers begins to change. The knee-jerk reaction gradually softens into a nonjudgmental response, and life is rendered far less stressful.

Two other major effects of consistent meditation practice are a deepening knowledge of the inner self and, perhaps, a direct experience of the awareness of that boundlessness that is the source of being and consciousness. Both of these experiences can open the individual's mind and heart to a feeling of unity and greater connection to the whole of life. It has been said that the language of the Infinite is silence. If so, we can hear that language only in stillness and silence. Not only does one's creativity come from this inner stillness, but the silence within is the deep well from which all of life arises.

In classical yoga theory and practice, meditation is a process of several steps:

· Holding one's total attention on an object of concentration (*Dhāraṇā*)
· Prolonging this attention until a relationship develops between the object of concentration and the mind (*Dhyāna*)
· Merging the object and the mind so that the mind sees the object as it is, without prior conditioning (*Samādhi*)

This process can be experienced with an object of attention or without an object of attention. With an object, one learns to view an object as it really is without making judgments based on past conditioning. The development of this ability is a valuable asset to the performer, who encounters many situations that have the potential to affect performance directly or indirectly. Meditation without an object is more related to experiencing union with one's inner self and with the Source of one's being.

Meditation Practices

There are numerous meditation techniques and practices that are valuable for various purposes. It is sometimes difficult to distinguish between concentration and meditation, and that is because they are two parts of the same phenomenon. Concentration precedes meditation and flows naturally into it; therefore, some practices seem to fall into both categories.

♦ *Focus on the Breath*

- Sitting with straight spine, head a little back, chin a little down, relaxed jaw, tongue, shoulders, and arms, eyes closed, bring your awareness to the breath at the tip of the nostrils
- Establish a smooth, flowing 6-count Inhalation/6-count Exhalation for 6 repetitions
- Keeping your focus on the breath at the nostrils, drop the counting and simply follow the natural movement of your breath
- When thoughts or feelings arise and your attention wanders, notice where your attention went, and gently, without judgment, return your awareness to the flow of the breath
- At first you may experience a "waterfall" effect of many thoughts and feelings rushing into your mind. Over time, as you continue to practice, the "waterfall" may slow to a flowing "river" of mental activity. The goal is to experience a "lake" effect—the mind is still like a calm lake with no movement on its surface. This will typically happen for only brief moments at a time, but the accumulation of these moments begins to effect a change in thought habits.

♦♦ *Use of "So-hum" or Other Mantra*

This is a repeated word, often of only one syllable, used as a focus of awareness.

"So" and "hum" are syllables said to represent the sounds of the inhalation and exhalation of the breath

- Sitting with a straight spine, relaxed shoulders, arms, hands, jaw, forehead muscles, eyes closed, lengthen your breath to a 6-count IN/ 6-count EX
- After 6 repetitions of the 6/6 breath, begin mentally to say, or hear, the mantra "So-hum": "Sooooooo" on the inhalation and "Huuuummmmm" on the exhalation, making the saying/thinking/hearing of each sound the entire length of the 6-count IN or EX; be totally present in the inner sound
- Strive for 12 repetitions of the mantra without losing your focus
- After 12 repetitions, follow the mantra in whatever way your mind works until you reach a moment of mental stillness and silence
- When your mind wanders, return gently and without judgment to the mantra
- This is a Concentration/Meditation practice that trains the mind to be one-pointed and leads into the stillness necessary for the silence of Contemplation

♦♦ "Big Sky" (thoughts as passing clouds)[3]

- Sit with a straight spine, relaxed shoulders, arms, hands, jaw, forehead muscles, eyes closed
- Look inward mentally and imagine a vast blue sky. It is all that you can see, as if you were lying on your back in a totally open space or floating freely and weightlessly in space. Be totally present to the blue sky
- Allowing your breath to find its natural rhythm, become absorbed in the vast blue sky
- As a thought or feeling arises, transform it into a cloud and watch the cloud float away until it vanishes and only the vast blue sky remains
- Remain absorbed in this image, watching cloud-thoughts come and go of their own accord, for some time

♦♦ Flowing River (thoughts as boats)[4]

- Sit with a straight spine, relaxed shoulders, arms, hands, jaw, forehead muscles, eyes closed
- Look inward mentally and imagine a flowing river; immerse your mind in the flow of the water
- As thoughts or feelings arise, transform them into boats floating down the river; allow each boat to float on past and out of sight without inspecting it or its cargo

- Remain absorbed in this image until there is more and more space between boats and your awareness is entirely in the flowing river

◆ ◆ ◆ *"Big Mind" (expansion from individual to edges of the universe)*[5]

- Sitting with straight spine, head a little back and chin a little down, relaxed forehead muscles, jaw, tongue, shoulders and arms, eyes closed, breathe normally but fully
- Focus your awareness just behind your forehead or in the center of your brain
- Successively and slowly, as guided, expand your awareness from each location to the next, including everything in the spaces
- All the space in your own skull—all the space in the room—all the space of your town—of your state or province—of your country—of the entire Earth—of our solar system—of our galaxy—of the billions of galaxies and trillions of stars—to the very edge of our expanding universe—to Infinity
- Rest in this space for a few breaths
- Now expand your heart around your mind in this enormous space
- Gradually bring your mind and heart back from Infinity through all the stars and interstellar spaces to our galaxy—our solar system—our blue planet—your country—your state or province—your town—this room—your own skull—your forehead center or heart center
- Lie back in *Śavāsana*, resting in your still mind and open heart

◆ *Metta (loving kindness meditation)*[6]

- Sit with a straight spine, relaxed shoulders, arms, hands, jaw, forehead muscles, eyes closed
- Bring your attention to your breath, flowing in and out in a long, smooth stream
- Turn your attention to your own care and well-being, as if you were your only child
- Say silently to yourself on breathing in, "May I be free from suffering," and on breathing out, "May I be at peace"; continue for some time
- Then bring to mind someone for whom you care deeply and say silently to that person on breathing in, "May you be free from suffering," and on breathing out, "May you be at peace"; continue for some time
- Now bring to mind someone for whom you have negative feelings and silently say to that person on breathing in, "May you be free from

suffering," and on breathing out, "May you be at peace"; continue for some time
- Finally, bring to mind all the living beings on earth and say silently on breathing in, "May all living beings be free from suffering," and on breathing out, "May all living beings be at peace"; continue for some time until your heart is at peace

♦ ♦ Contemplative Prayer (use of breath, religious icon, meaningful word or mental image as point of focus)

- Sit with a straight spine, relaxed shoulders, arms, hands, jaw, forehead muscles, eyes closed
- Using any focus that works for you, allow your mind to become still
- After some time, allow your awareness to sink into your heart; rest your mind on the flow of breath at the heart center
- Remain resting in your own heart for some time

6

Yoga and Singing

Both lead to the knowledge and expression of the soul.
They are natural partners.

Connections

The performer is a composite of voice, body, breath, mind, and heart. The singer must be at one with each of these facets of the person to put them all together into a single force.

Almost every conference address given by a professional opera director, an agent for singers, or others who are involved in the development of young professional singers makes reference to the "total package" needed for success. This phrase, which most likely comes from the marketing industry, refers to the singer who has all the gifts and abilities needed to be a versatile performer. Certainly those singers who advance to the status of young artists possess the basic equipment naturally—voice, musical ability, good looks, an agile mind—but the ability to use this basic equipment has been carefully trained over a long period of time. In the preceding chapters, we have explored how yoga practices train the body, the breath, the mind, and the heart. Let us now look at how the elements of a complete yoga practice complement and train the whole singer.

The Whole Singer

Command of the Body

The Whole Singer must first have command of the body as the singing instrument. The physical elements of posture and alignment, the muscles of the breathing mechanism, and the smooth functioning of the vocal mechanism itself are all elements that must be developed and trained. These elements are addressed in the yoga practices of *āsana* (physical postures) and *prāṇāyāma* (breathing practices, including humming). The coordination of movement with both breath and sound in metrical patterns reinforces many of the skills needed in actual singing.

The Whole Singer also needs command of the body as the acting instrument for stage performance. As the acting instrument, the body must be flexible and expressive to convey aspects of many different kinds of characters. The use of various arm adaptations in the physical postures builds strength and flexibility into the arms and hands for ease of gesture, and the standing postures build strength into the legs and torso for different types of stance and movement.

Command of the body as the vehicle of movement becomes increasingly necessary for the operatic or music theater singer who must work on sometimes improbable sets. One of the most difficult elements of modern staging is the raked stage, which seems to become ever steeper, especially for televised performance. Standing and moving for long periods on a raked stage is hard on the lower back, and the singer must develop strength in the lumbar and pelvic areas. Climbing steep flights of stairs requires strong quadriceps and a good sense of balance. Those postures that build strength in the legs, including leg balances, are excellent training for movement onstage.

Command of the body includes warming up the body before a performance and returning the body to normal after a performance with short practices that counteract strenuous actions on stage. It is also necessary to be able to relax the body for sleep after a performance, partially a function of mental relaxation.

Command of the Breath

The Whole Singer must have command of the breath, not only for singing but also as a constant focus of attention to which it is natural to return from any unexpected distraction. Unexpected things can and do happen on stage, and the natural reaction of the nervous system is to catch and hold the breath in such situations. It is vital to be able to keep the breath long and smooth as much as possible. The breathing practices of yoga train this ability.

Command of the breath includes the control of energy in performance. If the breath patterns are disrupted, the flow of energy is also disrupted. The word *prāṇā* means "vital energy" that is usually expressed as breath, an indication that the two are so closely related as to be seen as one thing. For this reason, the study and practice of the breath in yoga is also the study and practice of vital energy, the life force.

Command of the Mind

The Whole Singer must have command of the mind as the instrument of efficient learning and complete attention. The musical and acting demands of operatic singing in particular are such that learning an entire musical score, more often than not in a different language from one's own, and all the staging, not to mention creating a character, demand a highly efficient learning process. The concentration techniques of yoga train the mind to be both focused and free of distraction at will, skills that greatly aid learning and memorizing words, music, and movement. These practices further train the art of complete attention to the task at hand. The mind is also the instrument of overall coordination, of putting all the elements together into a seamless whole. The various combinations of movement, breath, and sound in *āsana* train the mind in the art of coordination.

The Whole Singer must have command of the mind as the instrument of attitude and behavior. It is easy to lose one's personal equilibrium under the stresses of intense rehearsal and performance. Training the mind to be non-judgmental is not only possible but necessary for the greatest success. This ability is gained through the concentration and meditation practices of yoga in which the mind is trained to allow thoughts and feelings to arise and disappear without reaction, judgment, or attachment. Where there is no judgment or attachment, equilibrium is far easier to maintain. This allows the singer to turn all the energy of passion into singing instead of wasting it in unskillful attitudes and behavior.

Communication with Heart and Soul

The Whole Singer must be in communion with his or her own heart and soul as the instruments of understanding, the sources of communication, and the places of presence in each moment. These aspects of the person are revealed and deepened through the practice of meditation that leads one inward to the self and the Source of all things.

Command of Relaxation

Finally, the Whole Singer must be able to relax mentally under extreme stress in order to use all the gifts and abilities to their highest potential. This ability to remain calm and balanced in all situations can be learned over time with the techniques of deep relaxation that condition the nervous system to function smoothly under stress.

Deep Relaxation Practices

◆ *Tension and Release*

· Lying in *Śavāsana*, observe your breathing for a moment
· Tense the muscles of your face and hold tightly for five seconds, then release
· Tense the muscles of your jaw, neck, and shoulders and hold tightly for five seconds, then release
· Continue tensing, holding, and releasing the muscles in the following areas of the body: arms, hands (make fists), chest and abdomen, hips and buttocks, thighs, calves, ankles, and feet
· Then tense all the muscles of the entire body, hold for five to ten seconds, and release
· Lie still for three to five minutes, allowing all your muscles to seem to melt into the floor; quietly observe your whole body breathing, completely relaxed—body, breath, and mind

◆ ◆ ◆ *31 or 61 Points*

This practice involves moving breath and awareness together from point to point throughout the body (*Śavayatra* or Traveling through the Body); *use upper half of body, lower half of body, or whole body, according to need.*

· Lying in *Śavāsana*, observe your breathing for a moment
· Allow stillness to arise in body and mind
· Gently bring your awareness to the center of your forehead
· Inhale 6 counts, keeping your awareness at the forehead center
· Exhale 6 counts, moving your awareness to the hollow of the throat
· Continue this 6-count Inhale/6-count Exhale pattern from point to point on your body, moving awareness and breath together, to the following points:
    · Right shoulder, elbow, wrist, thumb, tip of each finger separately, back to wrist, elbow, shoulder, and back to throat
    · Same points on left side, ending at the throat
    · To center of chest, solar plexus, navel center
    · Right hip, knee, ankle, big toe, other four toes separately, back to ankle, knee, hip, and back to navel center
    · Same points on left side, ending at navel center
    · Back to heart center, left side of chest, heart center, right side of chest, heart center

- Rest your breath at the heart center for some time, relaxing body, breath, and mind completely
- When you are ready, bring your awareness back to the room, move hands and feet, open your eyes, and come up to a sitting posture
- Remain sitting for a few moments before getting up

♦ ♦ ♦ Awareness of Light in the Body

- Lying in *Śavāsana,* observe your breathing for a moment
- Using the "61 or 31 Points" pattern above, move awareness of a point of light throughout the body, coordinated with the breath
- When you have finished, relax completely, feeling your whole body filled with light

♦ ♦ A Shorter Point-to-Point Awareness Relaxation

- Lying in *Śavāsana,* observe your breathing for a moment
- Begin with awareness at forehead center
- Inhale 6 at forehead center
- Exhale 6 to throat; Inhale 6
- Exhale 6 to center of chest; Inhale 6
- Exhale 6 to solar plexus; Inhale 6
- Exhale 6 to below navel; Inhale 6
- Exhale back to solar plexus, heart center, throat, forehead center
- Rest at forehead center—or heart center—for a few moments

Conclusion

In summary, the practice of yoga has many and broad-ranging benefits for the singer. The physical benefits include strengthening, developing, and conditioning the body as the singing instrument; extending and gaining control over all aspects of the breath; learning to relax under stress; promoting good health on all levels; and making it easier to move around in our vehicle for living. The mental benefits include learning how to develop a one-pointed mind useful for all types of concentrated attention, how to quiet the mind for mental rest and meditation, and how to let go of past conditioning and present distractions that interfere with confident performance. The emotional and spiritual benefits include learning meditation techniques that help to change unwanted habits of thought, speech, or action and form desirable habits that help to set a positive direction for the future; that expand the mind and heart;

and that take the person deep inside to discover the answer to the question, "Who am I?" In short, yoga practices work on refining the vehicle (the body) and the instrument (the mind) for the use of the deepest self. For the singer, the coordination of this totality frees the heart and spirit to sing.

Practices for Various Needs

Chart of *Āsanas* Especially Useful to the Developing Singer

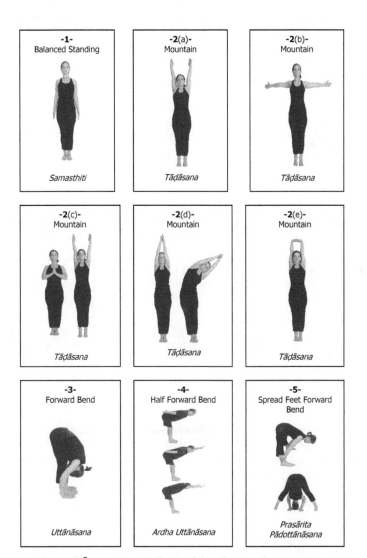

FIGURE II.I Chart of *Āsanas* Especially Useful to the Developing Singer [7 pages]

-6- Chair Posture	-7- Intense Side Stretch	-8- Half Intense Side Stretch
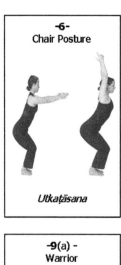	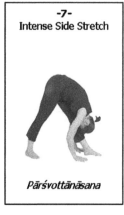	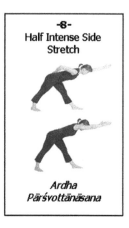
Utkaṭāsana	*Pārśvottānāsana*	*Ardha Pārśvottānāsana*

-9(a) - Warrior	-9(b)- Warrior	-9(c)- Warrior
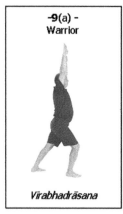	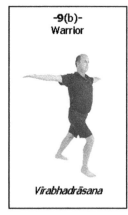	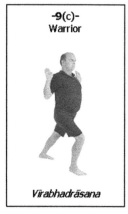
Vīrabhadrāsana	*Vīrabhadrāsana*	*Vīrabhadrāsana*

-10- Extended Triangle	-11- Extended Lateral Angle	-12- Revolved Triangle
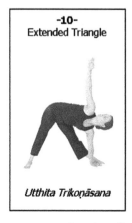	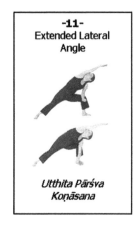	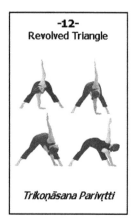
Utthita Trikoṇāsana	*Utthita Pārśva Koṇāsana*	*Trikoṇāsana Parivṛtti*

FIGURE II.I (continued)

-13- Mountain with Balance Variations (a) (b) 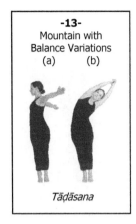 *Tāḍāsana*	-14- Tree 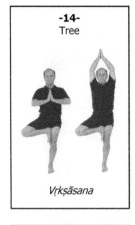 *Vṛkṣāsana*	-15- Standing Big Toe Holding Posture 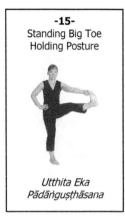 *Utthita Eka Pādāṅguṣṭhāsana*
-16- Warrior, Balance Variation 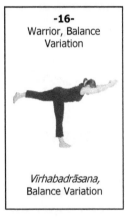 *Vīrhabadrāsana,* Balance Variation	-17- One-Footed Forward Bend 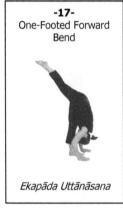 *Ekapāda Uttānāsana*	-18- Downward Facing Dog 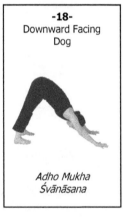 *Adho Mukha Śvānāsana*
-19- Ruddy Goose 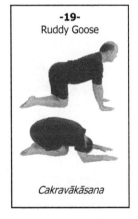 *Cakravākāsana*	-20- Kneeling Forward Bend 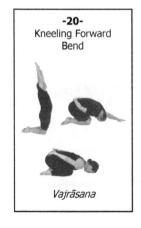 *Vajrāsana*	-21- One Footed Pigeon King with FB Variation 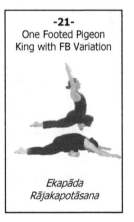 *Ekapāda Rājakapotāsana*

FIGURE II.I (continued)

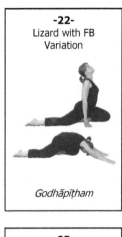

-22-
Lizard with FB
Variation

Godhāpīṭham

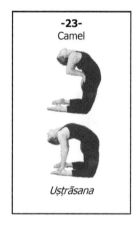

-23-
Camel

Uṣṭrāsana

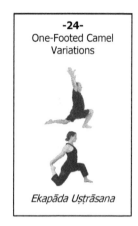

-24-
One-Footed Camel
Variations

Ekapāda Uṣṭrāsana

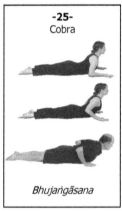

-25-
Cobra

Bhujaṅgāsana

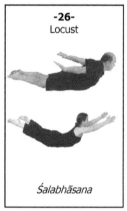

-26-
Locust

Śalabhāsana

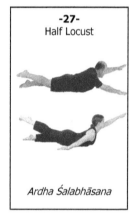

-27-
Half Locust

Ardha Śalabhāsana

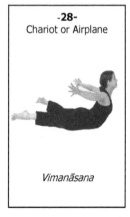

-28-
Chariot or Airplane

Vimanāsana

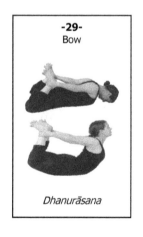

-29-
Bow

Dhanurāsana

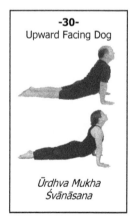

-30-
Upward Facing Dog

*Ūrdhva Mukha
Śvānāsana*

FIGURE II.I (continued)

170

-31- Upward Feet Posture	-32- Supine Big Toe Holding Posture	-33- Tank
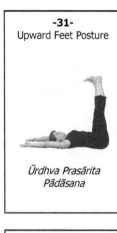	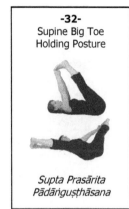	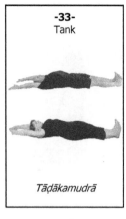
Ūrdhva Prasārita *Pādāsana*	*Supta Prasārita* *Pādāṅguṣṭhāsana*	*Tāḍākamudrā*

-34- Corpse	-35- Supine Bound Angle	-36- Supine Forward Bend
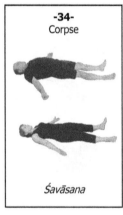	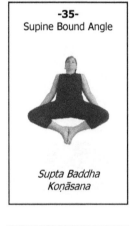	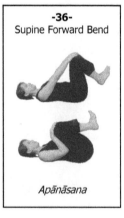
Śavāsana	*Supta Baddha* *Koṇāsana*	*Apānāsana*

-37- Bridge or Two-Footed Posture	-38- Supine Lateral Bend	-39- Supine Abdominal Twist
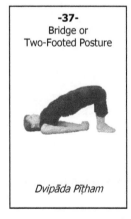	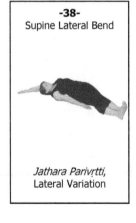	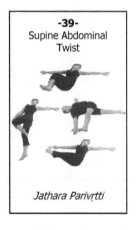
Dvipāda Pīṭham	*Jathara Parivṛtti,* Lateral Variation	*Jathara Parivṛtti*

FIGURE II.I (continued)

-40- Hero	-41- Easy Seated Posture	-42- Stick or Staff Posture
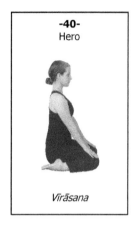	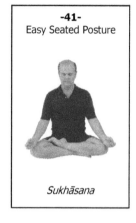	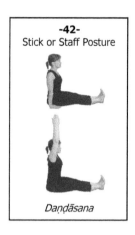
Vīrāsana	*Sukhāsana*	*Daṇḍāsana*
-43- Bound Angle	-44- Seated Forward Bend	-45- Boat
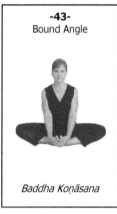	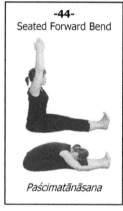	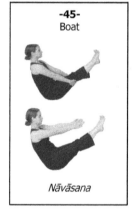
Baddha Koṇāsana	*Paścimatānāsana*	*Nāvāsana*
-46- Seated Triangle	-47- Head to Knee Posture	-48- Supine Hero
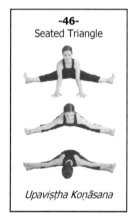	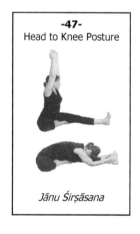	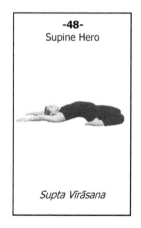
Upaviṣṭha Koṇāsana	*Jānu Śīrṣāsana*	*Supta Vīrāsana*

FIGURE II.I (continued)

-49- Easy Seated Twist	-50- Half Seated Twist	-51- Revolved Head to Knee
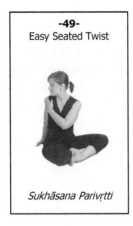	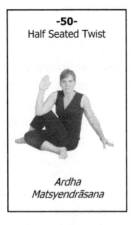	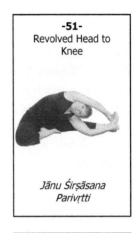
Sukhāsana Parivṛtti	*Ardha Matsyendrāsana*	*Jānu Śirṣāsana Parivṛtti*

-52- Inverted Posture	-53 Legs up the Wall	-54- Shoulderstand
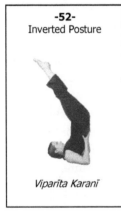	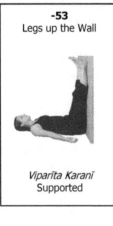	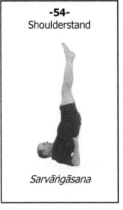
Viparīta Karanī	*Viparīta Karanī* Supported	*Sarvāṅgāsana*

-55- Plough	-56- Lion	-57- Eye Stretches See Instructions -58- Neck Stretches See Instructions
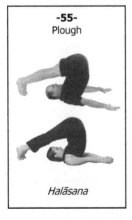	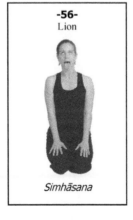	
Halāsana	*Simhāsana*	

FIGURE II.I (continued)

The practices in Part II are specific to various areas of the body, common problems of developing singers, and various situations for the performer. The numbers refer to the *Āsana* chart II.1 and to the numbered list in chapter 2 that gives information about and instructions for each posture. The sequences and various breathing and concentration practices are designed to be accessible to those who have experience with yoga and to those who are novices. They are by no means the only approaches to the designated use and can be adjusted to fit each individual need. The help of a knowledgeable teacher is always an advantage.

- Levels of difficulty are indicated before each practice: ♦ = Beginning; ♦ ♦ = Intermediate; ♦ ♦ ♦ = Advanced
- IN/EX = Inhale/Exhale; numbers refer to the number of counts per IN and EX; e.g., IN4/EX4 = 4-count IN/4-countEX; X = number of repetitions
- *Use IN4/EX4 breath throughout these sequences initially.* When comfortable with the 4/4 length, longer breath counts intensify the effects of each posture.
- The "stay" portion of a posture generally comes on the last repetition
- Always rest in *Śavāsana* at the end of each practice. Remember that in *Śavāsana* it is important for the arms to be slightly away from the torso and the palms facing upward in an open and receptive posture.

Sequences for Specific Areas of the Body

♦ *A Sequence to Strengthen Feet, Legs, Knees, and Ankles*

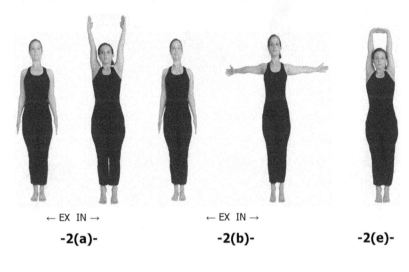

← EX IN →
-2(a)-

← EX IN →
-2(b)-

-2(e)-

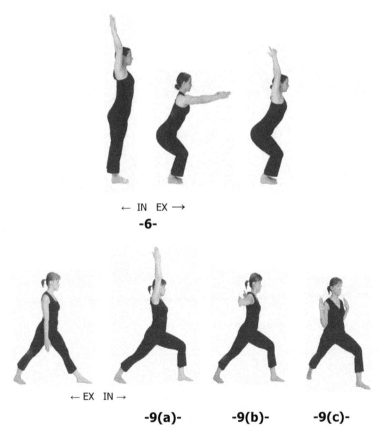

← IN EX →
-6-

← EX IN →
-9(a)-   **-9(b)-**   **-9(c)-**

FIGURE II.2   A Sequence to Strengthen Feet, Legs, Knees, and Ankles [2 pages]

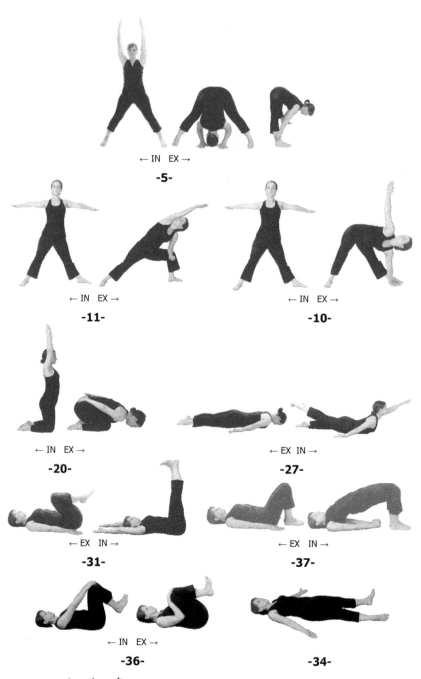

← IN EX →
-5-

← IN EX →
-11-

← IN EX →
-10-

← IN EX →
-20-

← EX IN →
-27-

← EX IN →
-31-

← EX IN →
-37-

← IN EX →
-36-

-34-

FIGURE 11.2 (continued)

- 2. Mountain with arm and heel raises: (a) x4; (b) x4; (e) stay 3 breaths with arm movements
- 6. Chair Posture: x4; stay 2, 4, 6, 8 counts
- 9. Warrior with arm variations: (a) x2; (b) x2; (c) x2; stay 2 breaths last time; repeat on opposite side
- 5. Spread Feet Forward Bend: x2; stay 4 breaths, lifting chest and straightening knees on IN, slightly bending knees and dropping top of head toward or to floor on EX
- 11. Extended Lateral Angle: x2 each side; stay 2–4 breaths
- 10. Extended Triangle: x2 each side; stay 2–4 breaths
- 20. Kneeling Forward Bend: x4
- 27. Half Locust: x2–4 alternate sides
- 31. Upward Feet Posture: x2; stay 2 breaths
- 37. Bridge or Two-Footed Posture: x4; stay 2–4 breaths last time
- 36. Supine Forward Bend: x4

◆ *A Sequence to Strengthen the Lower Abdominal Muscles*

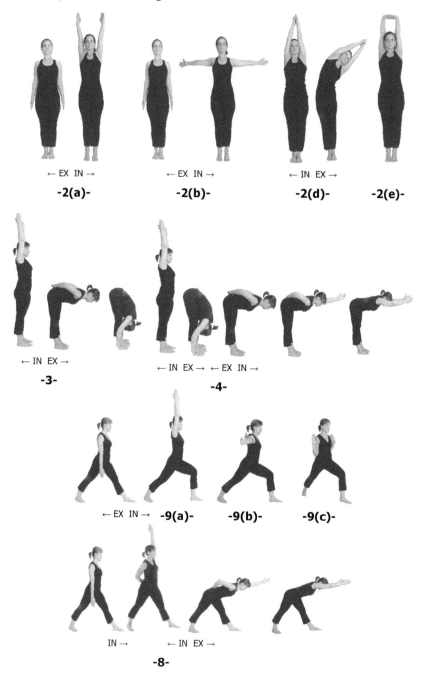

FIGURE 11.3 A Sequence to Strengthen the Lower Abdominal Muscles [2 pages]

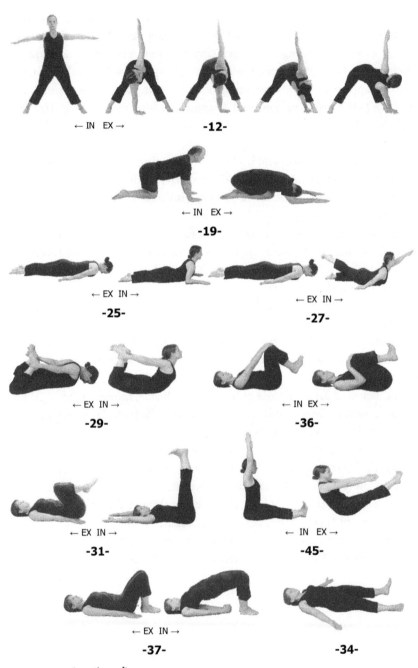

← IN EX →

-12-

← IN EX →

-19-

← EX IN →

-25-

← EX IN →

-27-

← EX IN →

-29-

← IN EX →

-36-

← EX IN →

-31-

← IN EX →

-45-

← EX IN →

-37-

-34-

FIGURE II.3 (continued)

All postures contribute to lower abdominal strength because the lower abdominal muscles are contracted when moving into and out of most postures, as well as during "stay" in many postures. The following sequence includes postures that work the abdominals while working other muscles also, and prepare for and compensate after the core poses. Core poses: 8. Half Intense Side Stretch, 12. Revolved Triangle, 29. Bow, and 45. Boat. Use IN4/EX4 for all postures.

- 2. Mountain with arm and heel raises, abdominal muscles contracted, breathe into ribs: (a) x4; (b) x4; (d) x2 alternate sides; (e) stay 3 breaths
- 3. Standing Forward Bend: x2 halfway with arms behind back; full bend, stay 2 breaths
- 4. Standing Half Forward Bend: from full bend, IN halfway up x4: arms behind, one arm forward, opposite arm forward, both arms forward; EX in position; IN to upright position; abdominal muscles remained contracted; IN into chest
- 9. Warrior: x6 each side, abdominals contracted; (a) x2; (b) x2; (c) x2; stay 2 breaths
- 8. Half Intense Side Stretch (core posture): x4 each side; arms behind, one arm forward; opposite arm forward; both arms forward and stay 2–4 breaths
- 12. Revolved Triangle (core posture): x4 each side, moving hand progressively from middle to outside of opposite foot; stay 2 breaths
- 19. Ruddy Goose (compensation): x4
- 25. Cobra: x4; stay 1–2 breaths last time
- 27. Half Locust: x2–4 alternate sides; stay 1 breath
- 29. Bow (core posture): x2; stay 2–4 breaths
- 36. Supine Forward Bend: x4; stay 4–6 counts after EX
- 31. Upward Feet Posture: x2; stay 2–4 breaths
- 45. Boat (core posture): stay 2–4 breaths (very strong abdominal work)
- 37. Bridge or Two-Footed Posture: x4; stay 2 breaths

♦ A Sequence to Stretch and Strengthen the Lower Back

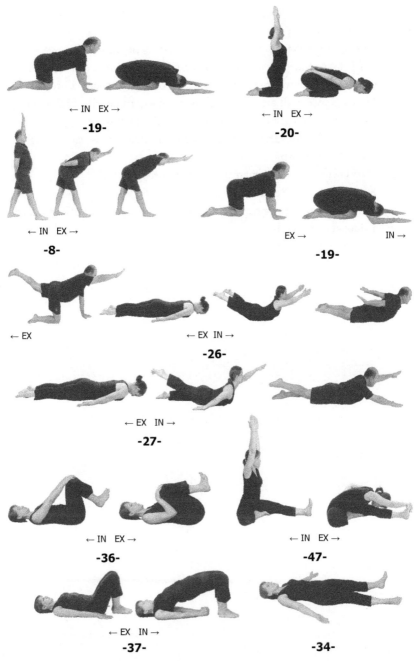

FIGURE 11.4 A Sequence to Stretch and Strengthen the Lower Back

To protect the lower back, *always* contract the lowest abdominal muscles to initiate movement into or out of a posture.

- 19. Ruddy Goose: x4
- 20. Kneeling Forward Bend: x4, sweeping arms behind back
- 8. Half Intense Side Stretch: x4 each side; arms behind back, one arm forward, opposite arm forward, both arms forward and stay 2 breaths
- 19. Ruddy Goose with arm and leg lifts: x4–6 alternate sides; IN, raising opposite arm and leg; EX back to Extended Child's Pose
- 26. Locust with arm variations: x2–4, arms on floor, arms back, arms forward; stay 2 breaths
- 27. Half Locust: x2–4 alternate sides; stay 1 breath
- 36. Supine Forward Bend (compensation): x4–6
- 47. Head to Knee with one arm back, other reaching to opposite foot: x2 each side; stay 2 breaths
- 37. Bridge or Two-Footed Posture (compensation): x4–6

♦ A Sequence to Stretch and Strengthen the Upper Back

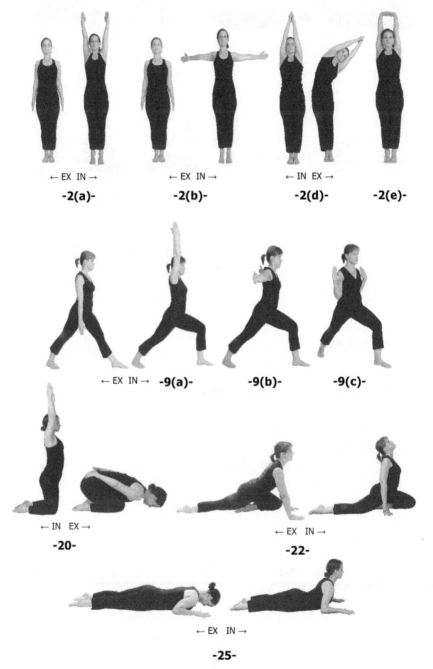

FIGURE II.5 A Sequence to Stretch and Strengthen the Upper Back [2 pages]

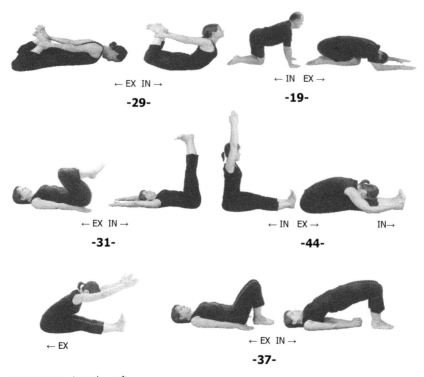

FIGURE 11.5 (continued)

- 2. Mountain with arm and heel raises: (a) x4; (b) x4; (d) x2 alternate sides; (e) stay 3 breaths
- 9. Warrior: x6 each side; (a) x2; (b) x2; (c) x2, stay 2–4 breaths
- 20. Kneeling Forward Bend: x4
- 22. Lizard: stay each side 2–4 breaths
- 25. Cobra with arm variations: x4; elbows on floor, elbows up, arms behind back, hands lifted off floor and stay 2 breaths
- 29. Bow: x2; stay 2–4 breaths
- 19. Ruddy Goose (compensation): x4
- 31. Upward Feet Posture: x2; stay 2–4 breaths
- 44. Seated Forward Bend with arm variation: x2; stay 2–4 breaths, leading with the chest, lift arms and torso to a 45-degree angle
- 37. Bridge or Two-Footed Posture: x4; stay 2–4 breaths

♦♦ A Sequence to Loosen and Strengthen the Neck and Shoulders

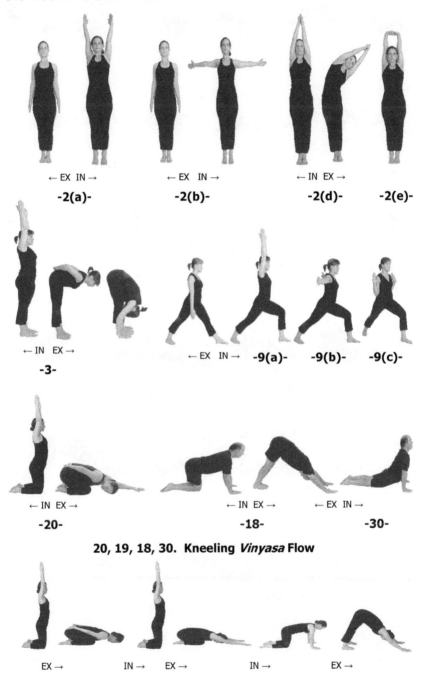

FIGURE 11.6 A Sequence to Loosen and Strengthen the Neck and Shoulders [2 pages]

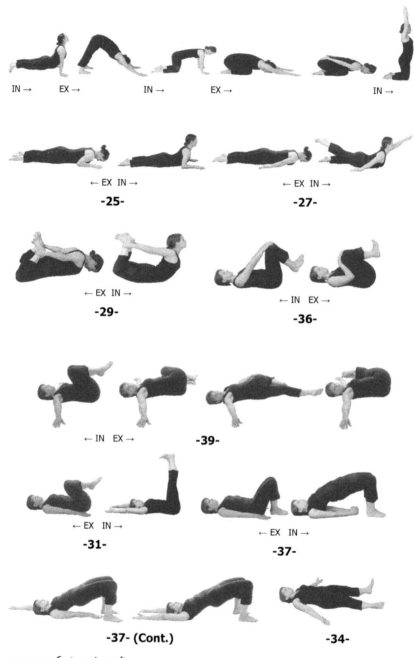

IN →   EX →   IN →   EX →   IN →

← EX IN →   ← EX IN →
-25-   -27-

← EX IN →   ← IN EX →
-29-   -36-

← IN EX →   -39-

← EX IN →   ← EX IN →
-31-   -37-

-37- (Cont.)   -34-

FIGURE II.6 (continued)

- 58. Neck Stretches: (see Instructions in Main *Āsana* List in chapter 2) stretch slowly and stay 1 breath in each position
- 2. Mountain sequence: (a) and (b) x4 each; (d) x2; (e) stay 3 breaths
- 3. Forward Bend: halfway x3, sweeping arms behind back; full bend, stay 4 breaths
- 9. Warrior: x6 each side with arm variations (a), (b), and (c), each x2; stay 2 breaths last time
- 20. Kneeling Forward Bend with head turns and alternating arms: x6
- 18. Downward Facing Dog: from hands and knees x2; stay 2–4 breaths
- 30. Upward Facing Dog: from Downward Facing Dog x4
- 20, 19, 18, 30. Kneeling *Vinyasa* Flow: each posture x2 ▶
- 25. Cobra: x4; stay 2 breaths last time
- 27. Half Locust: x2–4 alternate sides; stay 1 breath
- 29. Bow: x2; stay 2–4 breaths
- 36. Supine Forward Bend (compensation): x4
- 39. Supine Abdominal Twist with leg variations: x2 with bent knees; x1 with bent knee over straight leg; x1 straightening legs after twist
- 31. Upward Feet Posture: x2; stay 2—4 breaths
- 37. Bridge or Two-Footed Posture with arm variations: x4–6, alternating arms, then both arms

◆◆ A Sequence to Open and Strengthen the Hips

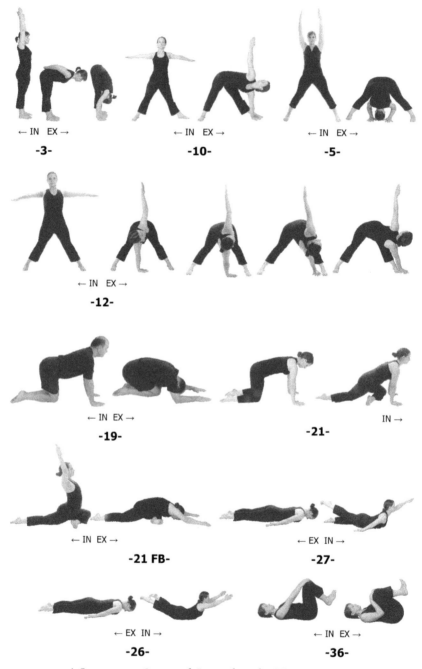

FIGURE 11.7 A Sequence to Open and Strengthen the Hips [2 pages]

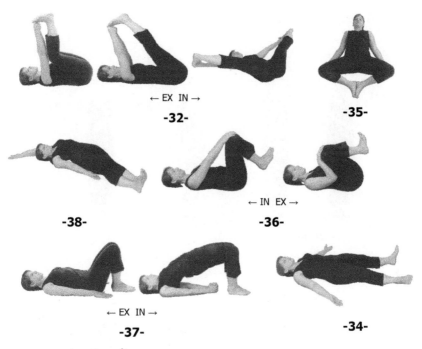

← EX IN →

-32-

-35-

-38-

← IN EX →

-36-

← EX IN →

-37-

-34-

FIGURE II.7 (continued)

- 3. Forward Bend: halfway x4, arms as desired; stay 2 breaths; full bend x2; stay 4 breaths
- 10. Extended Triangle: x2 each side; stay 2–4 breaths
- 5. Spread Feet Forward Bend: stay 2 breaths
- 12. Revolved Triangle: x4 each side, moving hand progressively; stay 2 breaths last time
- 19. Ruddy Goose (compensation): x4
- 21. One-Footed Pigeon King with forward bend variation: stay 2–4 breaths, folding forward over bent leg on last exhalation
- 27. Half Locust: x2–4 alternate sides
- 26. Locust: x2; stay 1 breath
- 36. Supine Forward Bend (compensation): x4–6
- 32. Supine Big Toe Holding with spread legs: stay with legs apart 2–4 breaths; close legs slowly, 8–20 counts x2
- 35. Supine Bound Angle: stay 2–4 breaths; close knees slowly, 8–20 counts x2
- 38. Supine Lateral Bend: stay 2–4 breaths each side
- 36. Supine Forward Bend (compensation): x4–6
- 37. Bridge or Two-Footed Posture: feet/knees together x2; gradually widen feet/knees x4

♦♦♦ A Sequence for Balance

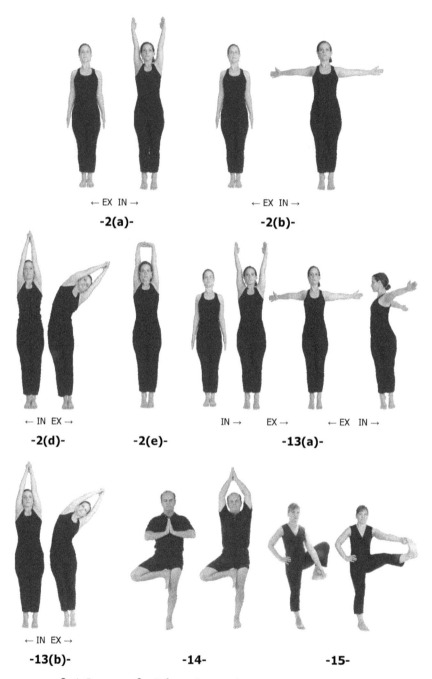

FIGURE 11.8 A Sequence for Balance [2 pages]

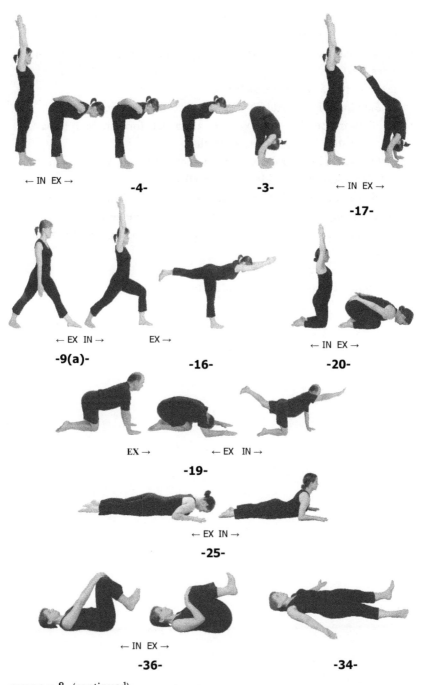

← IN EX →

-4-

-3-

← IN EX →

-17-

← EX IN →   EX →

-9(a)-

-16-

← IN EX →

-20-

EX →   ← EX IN →

-19-

← EX IN →

-25-

← IN EX →

-36-

-34-

FIGURE II.8 (continued)

- 2. Mountain sequence (warm-up): (a) and (b) x4 each; (d) x2 alternate sides; (e) stay 3 breaths
- 13. Mountain toe balance variations: (a) x2 alternate sides; (b) x1 alternate sides
- 14. Tree: stay 2–4 breaths each side
- 15. Standing Big Toe Holding: stay 2–4 breaths each side
- 4.3. Forward Bend: halfway x3, arms alternately forward, both forward, stay 2 breaths; full bend, stay 4 breaths
- 17. One-Footed Forward Bend: stay 2–4 breaths each side
- 9. Warrior: (a) x2 each side; stay 2 breaths
- 16. Warrior, Balance Variation: stay 2–4 breaths each side
- 20. Kneeling Forward Bend: x2 (symmetrical compensation)
- 19. Ruddy Goose with arm and leg lifts: x6, alternating opposite arm and leg lifts
- 25. Cobra: x4; stay 2 breaths
- 36. Supine Forward Bend (compensation): x4

A Complete Basic Practice for Daily Use

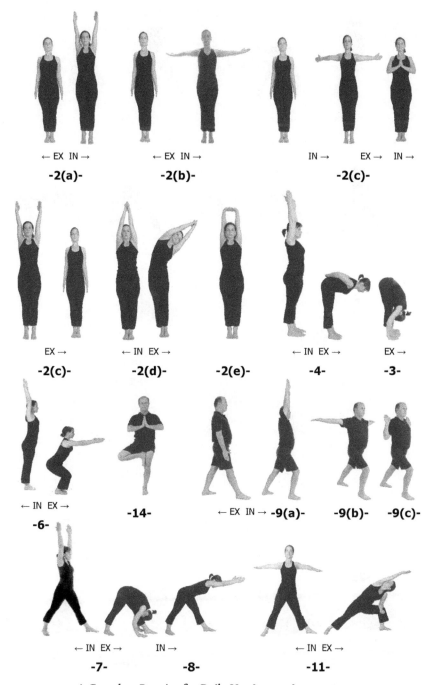

FIGURE 11.9 A Complete Practice for Daily Use [3 pages]

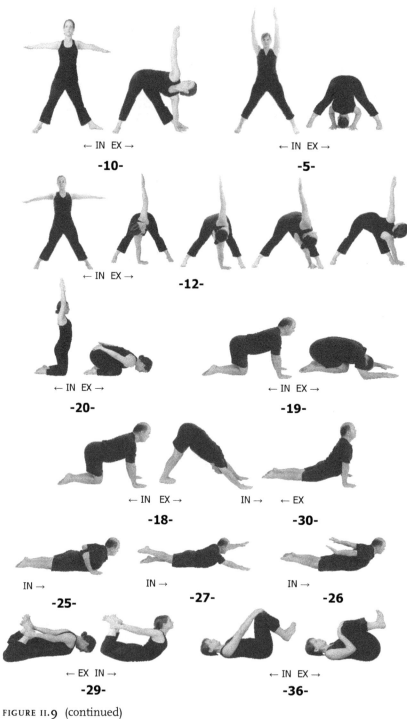

← IN EX →

-10-

← IN EX →

-5-

← IN EX →

-12-

← IN EX →

-20-

← IN EX →

-19-

← IN EX →

-18-

IN →   ← EX

-30-

IN →

-25-

IN →

-27-

IN →

-26

← EX IN →

-29-

← IN EX →

-36-

FIGURE II.9 (continued)

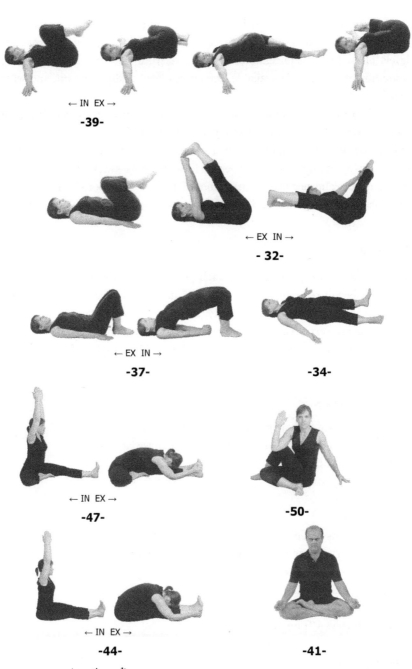

← IN EX →

-39-

← EX IN →

- 32-

← EX IN →

-37-   **-34-**

← IN EX →

-47-   **-50-**

← IN EX →

-44-   **-41-**

FIGURE II.9 (continued)

This complete practice includes a basic *āsana* practice that contains all positions and all directions of movement with beginning and intermediate levels of postures. Choices should be made from this practice, depending upon how much time is available, the energy level of the moment, and what will follow the practice.

In choosing postures for a sequence, the rule of thumb is to include one or two (or several, depending upon time) postures from all positions and directions and to use forward bending postures to transition between postures in other directions (for example, backward bend—forward bend—twist—forward bend—lateral bend). The postures chosen should address any specific structural or muscular concerns with care. Do not overdo the *āsana* portion of your practice.

I. Āsana

Choose one or two postures from each position and direction, a breath pattern, number of repetitions, and length of stay for each posture to suit your needs of the moment. Keep the order of positions from standing to seated unless you are very tired and wish to reverse the order and begin with supine postures and work up to standing. If you plan to do a long breathing practice, do a shorter physical practice to conserve energy.

Standing Postures

- ◆ 2. Mountain with arm and heel raises
- ◆◆ 4. Standing Half Forward Bend with arm variations
- ◆ 3. Forward Bend
- ◆ 6. Chair Posture
- ◆◆ 14. Tree
- ◆ 9. Warrior
- ◆◆ 7. Intense Side Stretch with arm variations
- ◆◆ 8. Half Intense Side Stretch with arm variations
- ◆◆ 11. Extended Lateral Angle
- ◆ 10. Extended Triangle
- ◆ 5. Spread Feet Forward Bend
- ◆ 12. Revolved Triangle

Kneeling Postures

- ◆ 20. Kneeling Forward Bend
- ◆ 19. Ruddy Goose
- ◆ 18. Downward Facing Dog
- ◆◆ 30. Upward Facing Dog

Prone Postures

- ◆ 25. Cobra
- ◆◆ 27. Half Locust
- ◆ 26. Locust
- ◆◆ 29. Bow

Supine Postures

- ◆ 36. Supine Forward Bend
- ◆ 39. Supine Abdominal Twist
- ◆◆ 32. Supine Big Toe Holding Posture
- ◆ 37. Bridge
- ◆ 34. Corpse

Seated Postures

- ◆◆ 47. Seated Head to Knee
- ◆◆ 50. Half Seated Twist
- ◆◆ 44. Seated Forward Bend
- ◆ 41. Easy Seated Posture

II. Prānāyāma

Choose a breathing practice for your needs of the moment

III. Concentration/Meditation

- Follow the breath to quiet the mind 3–5 minutes
- Then choose a practice that suits your needs of the moment

IV. Deep Relaxation

- Lie quietly in *Śavāsana* for a few moments, totally relaxing body, breath, and mind
- Or choose a particular practice that suits your needs of the moment

Short Practices for Specific Vocal Deficiencies

Always rest in *Śavāsana* at the end of a sequence. For seated practices, a "relaxed body" refers to relaxed shoulders, arms, jaw, and tongue.

Posture and Alignment

♦ Slumped chest

Use IN4/EX4 for all postures

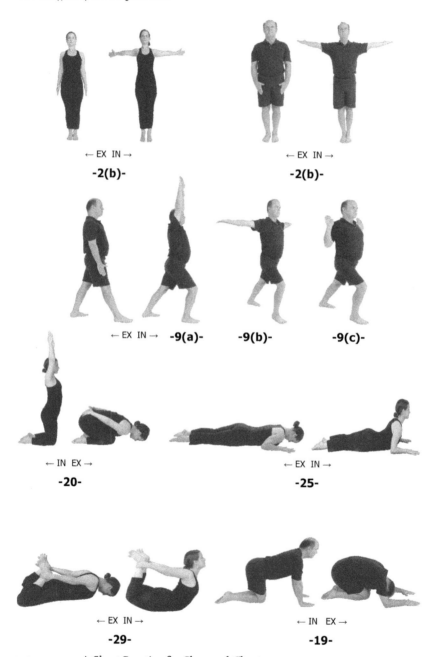

FIGURE 11.10 A Short Practice for Slumped Chest

- 2. Mountain with arm and heel raises: (b) x6; stay 2 breaths to open chest
- 9. Warrior: x6 each side, with arm variations to strengthen upper back muscles; stay 2–4 breaths last time
- 20. Kneeling Forward Bend: x4; transition to prone postures
- 25. Cobra: x4; stay 2 breaths to strengthen upper back and lower abdominal muscles
- 29. Bow; x2; stay 4 breaths to stretch front of body, shoulders, quadriceps, and strengthen upper back and lower abdominals
- 19. Ruddy Goose: x4; stay in Child's Pose 2–4 breaths

♦ Forward jutting chin

Use IN4/EX4 for all postures

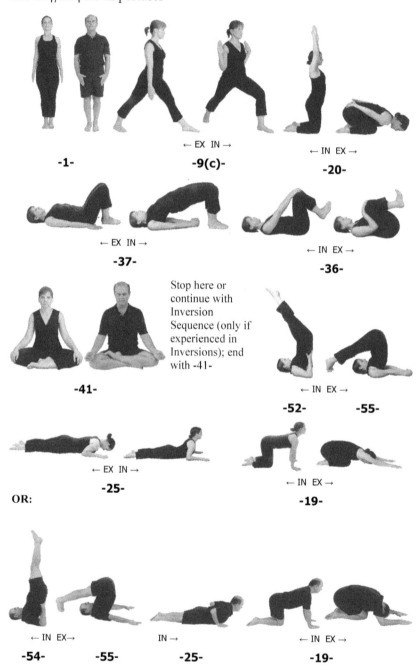

FIGURE II.II A Short Practice for Forward Jutting Chin

- 1. Balanced Standing Posture: with chin lock engaged, stay 4–6 breaths, to bring head in line with spine and stretch back of neck
- 9. Warrior: (c) x4; engage chin lock and stay 4–6 breaths to work upper back muscles, bring head in line with spine, and stretch back of neck
- 20. Kneeling Forward Bend: x4 keeping chin tucked; transition to supine postures
- 37. Bridge or Two-Footed Posture: x6; with chin tucked, stay 2–4 breaths to stretch back of neck
- 36. Supine Forward Bend: x4; compensation for backward bends
- 41. Easy Seated Posture: stay 4–8 breaths with chin lock to keep back of neck stretched during conscious breathing (*end sequence here* unless you are an experienced yoga practitioner or working with a teacher)
  - ◆ ◆ ◆ *(Optional: Continue only if an advanced yoga student with no contraindications)*
- 52. Inverted Posture or
- 54. Shoulderstand: stay 1–3 minutes to stretch back of neck and strengthen whole body
- 55. Plough: Stay a few moments; do not overstretch the back of the neck
- 25. Cobra: x4 to compensate for Shoulderstand and Plough
- 19. Ruddy Goose: x4; stay in Child's Pose 2–4 breaths

◆◆ Forward rolling shoulders
Use IN4/EX4 for all postures ⊚

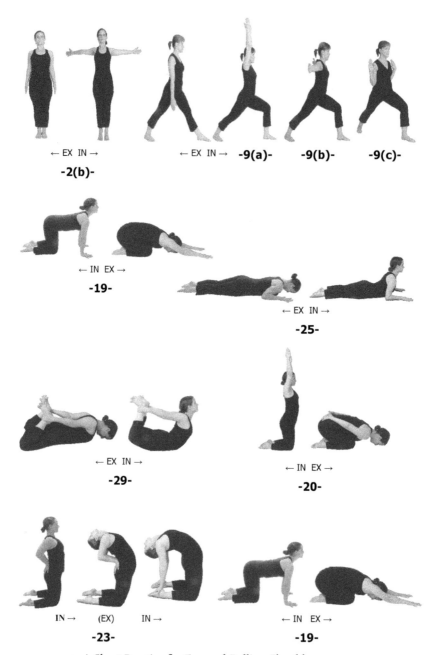

FIGURE 11.12 A Short Practice for Forward Rolling Shoulders

- 2. Mountain: with arm raises: (b) x4; stay 4 breaths to open the chest, pull shoulder blades together and down and shoulders back and down
- 9. Warrior: x6 each side, with arm variations; stay 2–4 breaths in (c) to strengthen shoulder blade muscles
- 19. Ruddy Goose: x4 lifting sternum up and forward on IN
- 25. Cobra: x4—2 with elbows on floor, 2 with elbows up; stay 1 breath to engage back muscles
- 29. Bow: x2; stay 1–4 breaths to stretch front of torso and deepen backward bend
- 20. Kneeling Forward Bend: x2 as compensation for backward bending
- 23. Camel: stay 2–6 breaths to stretch front of torso, shoulders, and open the chest
- 19. Ruddy Goose: x4; stay in Child's Pose 2-4 breaths

♦ Neck, shoulder, and arm tension

Use IN4/EX4 for all postures

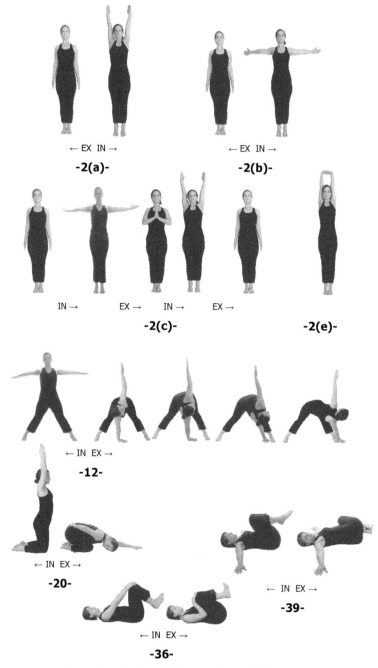

← EX IN →

-2(a)-

← EX IN →

-2(b)-

IN →   EX →   IN →   EX →

-2(c)-   **-2(e)-**

← IN EX →

-12-

← IN EX →

-20-

← IN EX →

-39-

← IN EX →

-36-

FIGURE 11.13 A Short Practice for Neck, Shoulder, and Arm Tension

- 2. Mountain with arm and heel raises: (a) x4; (b) x4; (c) x2; (e) stay 3 breaths
- 12. Revolved Triangle: x4 each side, moving hand progressively closer to opposite foot; stay 2 breaths in full rotation
- 20. Kneeling Forward Bend; x6; with head turns, alternating arms
- 39. Supine Abdominal Twist: x4–6 each side; with bent legs; stay 2–4 breaths last time each side
- 36. Supine Forward Bend: x4–6; compensation for twisting

♦ ♦ Uneven stance

Use IN4/EX4 for all postures

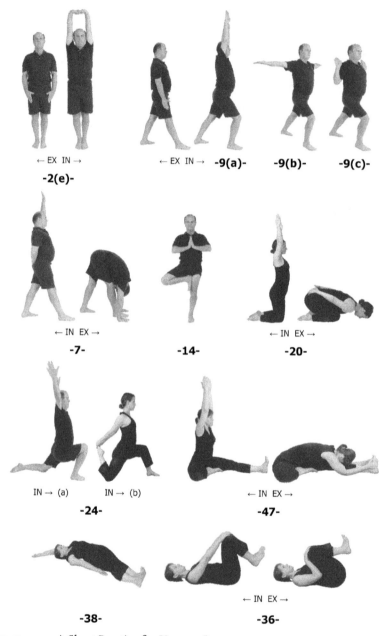

← EX IN →

-2(e)-

← EX IN →   -9(a)-   -9(b)-   -9(c)-

← IN EX →

-7-   -14-   -20-

IN → (a)   IN → (b)   ← IN EX →

-24-   -47-

-38-   ← IN EX →

                        -36-

FIGURE II.14 A Short Practice for Uneven Stance

- 2. Mountain: (e) x2; stay 2–4 breaths
- 9. Warrior: x6 each side with arm variations; stay 2 breaths on each side for working alternate sides of the body independently to see whether there is an imbalance in leg muscles
- 7. Intense Side Stretch: x4 each side; stay 2–4 breaths for working each side independently
- 14. Tree: stay 4–8 breaths each side to see whether there is an imbalance and to strengthen both sides
- 20. Kneeling Forward Bend: x4; symmetrical compensation
- 24. One Footed Camel Variations: (a) x2; stay 1 breath to stretch psoas muscle in straight leg; (b) stay 1–2 breaths to stretch front thigh muscles more deeply
- 47. Seated Head to Knee: x4 each side; stay 2–4 breaths last time
- 38. Supine Lateral Bend: stay 4–6 breaths each side, pushing heels out and using arm variation for stretching the front of the hip and the rib cage of each side of the body
- 36. Supine Forward Bend: x4; symmetrical compensation

♦ Locked knees

Use IN4/EX4 for all postures

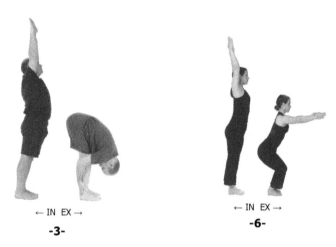

← IN EX →

-3-

← IN EX →

-6-

FIGURE 11.15   A Short Practice for Locked Knees

- 3. Standing Forward Bend with bent knees: x4; stay 2–4 breaths keeping knees slightly bent to release hamstrings
- 6. Chair Posture: x4; stay 2, 4, 6, 8 counts in succeeding repetitions

♦ Swayed back

Alternate stretching and contracting of the back muscles help to stretch the tight muscles of the lower back that contribute to a swayed back (lordosis): Use IN4/EX4

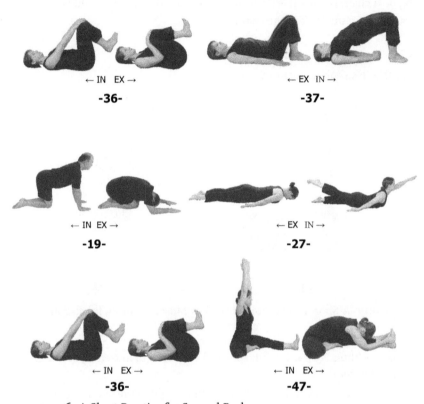

FIGURE 11.16 A Short Practice for Swayed Back

- 36. Supine Forward Bend: x6; stay2–4 breaths to gently stretch the lower back
- 37. Bridge or Two-Footed Posture: x6; stay 2–6 breaths to contract muscles of the lower back
- 19. Ruddy Goose: x6; stay 2–4 breaths to stretch the lower back
- 27. Half Locust: x4 on alternate sides to contract the muscles of the lower back
- 36. Supine Forward Bend: x4; stay 2–4 breaths to stretch the lower back
- 47. Seated Head to Knee: x2; stay 2–4 breaths each side to stretch alternate sides of the lower back

Breath Control

Many practices for breath control are seated practices. Always sit with straight spine, relaxed body (meaning relaxed shoulders, arms, jaw, tongue, and forehead muscles), and closed eyes. Any seated posture that is comfortable, including on a chair, is workable. If sitting on a chair, the spine should be erect and not touching the back of the chair.

♦ Neck muscles tense during inhalation
Use IN4/EX4 for all postures

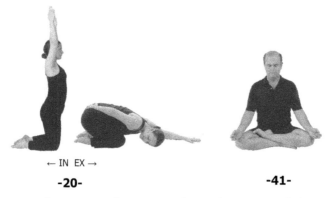

← IN EX →

-20-   **-41-**

FIGURE 11.17 A Short Practice for Tense Neck Muscles During Inhalation

- 20. Kneeling Forward Bend: x8 with head turns to loosen neck muscles and shoulders
- 41. Easy Seated Posture: (1) Sitting with straight spine and relaxed body, IN4 while turning head slowly to the left; EX4 while turning head back to center; repeat, turning head to the right; repeat x4–8, paying attention to keeping neck, shoulder, and jaw muscles relaxed; (2) Do a 4:4:4:4 ratio practice (see chapter 3), keeping neck, shoulders, jaw, and tongue relaxed

♦ ♦ Insufficient inhalation

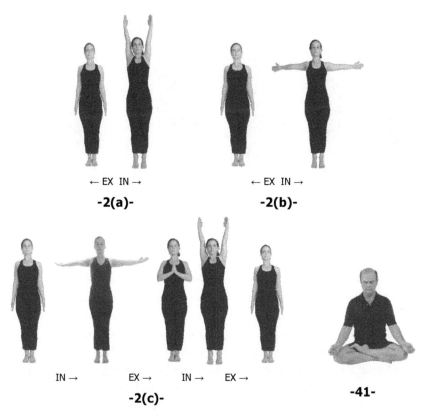

FIGURE 11.18 A Short Practice for Insufficient Inhalation

- 2. Mountain with arm and heel raises: (a) IN4/EX4 x4; (b) IN6/EX6 x4; (c) IN8/EX8 x2; (IN and arm motion for entire count)
- 41. Easy Seated Posture: Sitting with straight spine, relaxed body, do the following Ratio practice (may be done with alternate nostril technique): IN4/EX4 x4; IN4/SF2/EX4/SE2 x2; 4:4:4:4 x4; 6:4:6:4 x2; 6:6:6:6 x4; IN6/EX6 x2; IN4/EX4 x4; return to normal breathing and rest

♦ ♦ Breathy tone

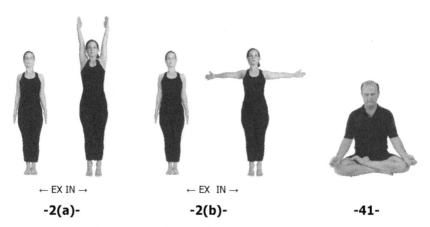

← EX IN →   ← EX IN →

-2(a)-   **-2(b)-**   **-41-**

FIGURE 11.19 A Short Practice for Breathy Tone

- 2. Mountain with arm and heel raises: (a) IN4/EX8, *Humming* a single pitch *pianissimo* (*pp*), focusing attention at the bridge of the nose, and using the smallest stream of breath possible (make the hum and the arm movement end at the same time) x2; (b) IN4/EX8 as before x2
- 41. Easy Seated Posture: Sitting with straight spine, relaxed body, IN4/EX4 x4; IN4 /engage root lock (see chapter 3), *Hum* single pitch (*pp*) 6 counts x4; IN4/engage root lock, *Hum* single pitch (*pp*) 8 counts x4; rest briefly and repeat the practice, being sure to keep root lock engaged throughout the humming

♦ Loss of breath during phrase

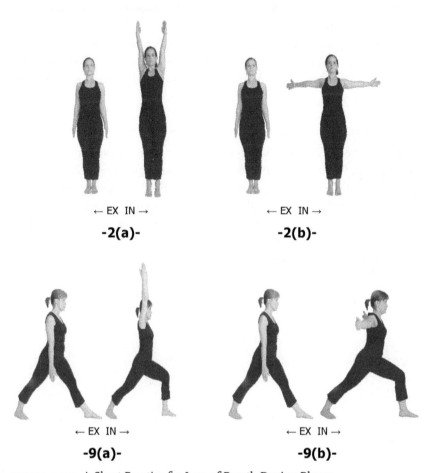

← EX IN →
-2(a)-

← EX IN →
-2(b)-

← EX IN →
-9(a)-

← EX IN →
-9(b)-

FIGURE 11.20 A Short Practice for Loss of Breath During Phrase

· 2. Mountain with arm and heel raises: (a) IN4/EX6 x2; IN4/EX8 x2; (b) IN4/EX10 x2; IN4/EX12 x2; pay attention to the smoothness of arm motion
· 9. Warrior: (a) IN4/EX6 x2; IN4/EX8 x2; (b) IN4/EX10 x2; IN4/EX12 x2, each side; pay attention to the smoothness of arm motion
· Gives too much at beginning: notice where you run out of breath; notice the speed of your arm motion. Do you move too fast at the beginning of the movement? If so, you also give too much breath at the beginning of the phrase

- Stops breath at some point: notice where your arms slow or stop movement during EX; notice your breath at these points. Where your arms change speed or stop is also where you tend to stop your breath during the phrase
- Stops saying the vowel sound of a long tone: Practice the two postures with a hum and vowel sounds. Notice where your arms tend to slow down or stop; this is where you also tend to stop saying the vowel sound during a long tone

♦ Abdominal muscles too tight on inhalation

- 41. Easy Seated Posture: Sitting with straight spine, relaxed body, IN4/EX4; IN completely into the belly, beginning with relaxed lower abdominal muscles; EX by gently pulling in the lower abdominal muscles and keeping the chest up and open x4; IN6, half into the belly and half into the chest, spreading the lower ribs/EX6 as before x4; IN8, half into the chest, spreading the lower ribs, and half into the belly/EX8 as before x4. Rest and repeat the practice

♦♦ Abdominal muscles pulled in too quickly during phrase

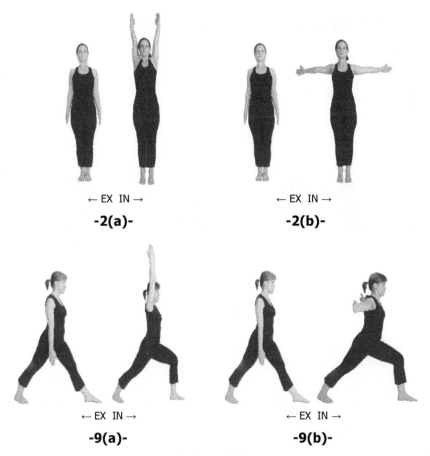

FIGURE II.21 A Short Practice for Smooth Abdominal Action

· 2. Mountain with arm raises only: (a) IN4, half into chest, spreading
  lower ribs, half into belly/EX8 x4; (b) IN4 as before/EX12 x4
· 9. Warrior: (a) IN4, half into chest, half into belly/EX8 x2; (b) IN4, as
  before/EX12 x2; repeat on opposite side.
· *In both postures*
· *Notice* the beginning of the EX and downward arm movement
· *Focus on* the very beginning of the EX and see how slowly you can begin a
  very narrow stream of breath felt at the highest point on the bridge of the
  nose, how slowly you can engage the lower abdominal muscles, and how
  slowly you can begin the arm movement downward

- Repeat postures using a Hum on the EX; find the precise point of balance between vibration (tone) and breath flow coordinated with downward arm movement.
- Repeat, using closed vowel sounds [i] or [e]

Mental Focus

♦♦ Lack of focus during lesson

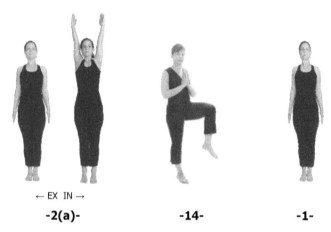

← EX IN →

-2(a)-   -14-   -1-

FIGURE 11.22 A Short Practice for Lack of Focus During the Private Lesson

- 2. Mountain: (a) IN4/EX4, 6, 8, 10, 12, slowly lowering arms and heels; focus eyes on one spot; focus attention on the feeling of arm movement and breath flow
- 14. Tree (Variation): with one knee raised parallel to the floor and hands together at chest, focus eyes on one spot; stay 2–4 breaths; repeat on opposite side
- 1. Balanced Standing Posture: Stand with eyes closed; focus on the feeling of breath flowing inside the nostrils; visualize the music at hand on the page. This is a good sequence to practice before a lesson if the mind is distracted.

♦ Loss of attention during performance
- 41. Easy Seated Posture: Sit with straight spine, relaxed body, closed eyes;
- Focus on the sensations of the flow of the breath inside the nostrils
- As thoughts or feelings arise, notice what they are—each one—and gently return your focus to the sensations of the breath

- After 5 minutes or so, visualize yourself performing. As distracting thoughts or feelings arise, name each one twice ("thinking, thinking"; "fear, fear"; "remembering, remembering," etc.) and gently return attention to the sensations of the breath in the nostrils
- After 5 minutes or so, hear yourself singing a specific song or aria; become completely absorbed in the experience; when distractions arise, name each one twice and return attention to the singing
- Do this practice every day for a month. Continue the practice as long as necessary to notice a difference in your performance focus.

♦ Constant mental distractions

- 41. Easy Seated Posture: Sitting with straight spine, relaxed body, closed eyes, focus on the sensations of the flow of breath inside the nostrils
- Lengthen the breath to IN6/EX6; complete 6 breaths without losing your focus
- As thoughts, feelings, memories, plans, or outside distractions arise, name each one twice ("thinking, thinking," etc.) and gently return your attention to the sensation of the breath flowing inside the nostrils
- This is a practice in letting go of mental distractions and returning to a focus
- Using a timer, begin with 5 minutes twice a day for 7 days
- Increase to 10 minutes twice a day for 7 days
- Increase to 15 minutes once a day for 7 days
- Increase to 20 minutes once a day for 7 days
- Notice whether your mental focus is more stable
- Continue the practice at the 10- or 15-minute level as a part of your daily activity

Difficulty in memorizing music: Two approaches

·   ◆ ◆ With a partner: memorizing by hearing and movement

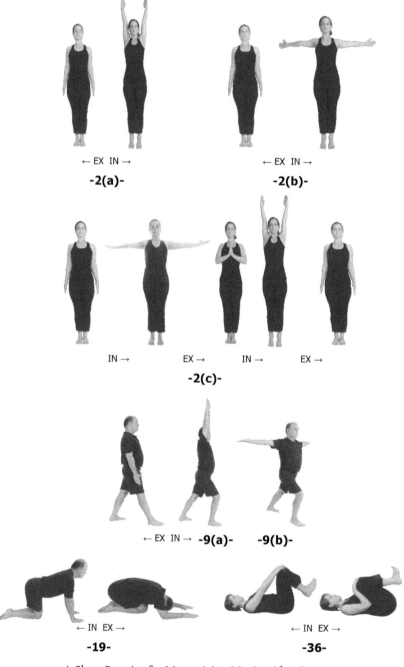

FIGURE 11.23 A Short Practice for Memorizing Music with a Partner

- Postures that are easy to use for this practice
  - 2. Mountain (a), (b), and (c)
  - 9. Warrior (a) and (b)
  - 19. Ruddy Goose
  - 36. Supine Forward Bend
- With a partner who knows the song or can read it from the score and using the length of IN and EX that corresponds to the phrase length
  - On IN, *listen* to partner sing first phrase while moving in the appropriate direction in the posture
  - On EX, *sing* the phrase while moving on the EX part of the posture
  - Repeat x2–3
  - Move to second phrase; repeat the process
  - Continue until you have finished the song
  - Use whichever posture is easiest for you; try different postures
  - The connection to movement assists focus and memory
- ♦ Working alone: memorizing by visualization (have music in front of you)
  - 41. Easy Seated Posture (or sit on a straight chair): Sitting with straight spine, relaxed body, eyes closed
    - Lengthen the breath to a IN6/EX6 x6, focusing on the sensations of the breath flowing inside the nostrils
    - On IN (adjust length of IN/EX to the length of the phrase), *look* at the first phrase, hearing it mentally
    - On EX *sing* the phrase mentally, looking at the notes
    - On IN look at phrase, hearing it mentally
    - On EX sing phrase mentally with eyes closed, visualizing it mentally
    - On IN *hear* the phrase mentally
    - On EX *sing phrase mentally* without visualizing notes
    - Repeat sequence for each phrase of song or aria
    - Connection to conscious breathing assists focus and memory; seeing, visualizing, and mentally hearing each phrase on the inhalation subconsciously brings the phrase into body, breath, mind, and heart and thus into the memory

Presence in Singing

The quality of presence in singing seems to be innate in some singers, somewhat evident in others, and totally lacking in a few otherwise fine singers. This quality is deeply connected to the singer's self-acceptance and joy in living.

It is a spiritual quality that can be developed, or released, in several ways. Yoga offers many practices for the acceptance and development of the self.

♦ No sense of personal presence

This phenomenon usually indicates a lack of connection to one's own emotions or a fear of losing control if the emotions touched by text or music are allowed to surface or come into play in singing. The singer with this problem probably needs some type of psychiatric help or counseling, as the lack of presence in singing may manifest in various other ways in daily life. However, there are meditation practices that help to connect to and accept buried or repressed feelings. A simple one is the following:

- 41. Easy Seated Posture: Sit comfortably and quietly, spine straight, body relaxed, eyes closed
- Bring your awareness to the breath; feel the whole body breathe
- Focus your awareness on the sensations of the breath flowing inside the nostrils
- Lengthen the breath to IN6/EX6 x6
- Bring to mind your singing and how you feel about it
- Name each thought and each emotion that arises and stay with each one, accepting its presence until it disappears of its own accord
- Accept whatever emotion appears as natural and healing; allow each one to run its course and disappear
- This is a practice in letting things surface in a safe way; if the experience is overwhelming, seek a person whom you trust and who understands the practice to be with you during this practice
- Repeat this practice daily for whatever length of time is possible until you begin to feel a change in your singing

♦♦ Overacting or inappropriate expressions and/or gestures

Overacting is sometimes a substitute for inner conviction. If this is the case, a practice for internalizing the elements of communication may be helpful.

- 41. Easy Seated Posture: Sit comfortably and quietly, spine straight, body relaxed, eyes closed
- Focus your awareness on the sensations of breath flowing inside the nostrils for a few moments to quiet your mind
- Bring to mind a particular song or aria in which you tend to overact
- In two or three words, name the emotions or meanings to be communicated

- Continue your focus on the breath for a few moments as you allow yourself to become each emotion or meaning—feeling each one in your whole body
- Now mentally sing the song or aria, feeling the emotion and meaning well up inside your body—motion in stillness
- Mentally sing the song or aria again, visualizing yourself using only half the external movement and gestures growing out of your internalization
- Stand and sing the song or aria; notice any difference in your communication
- Repeat this practice with each one of your songs and arias until you feel a real change in your performance

Performance Anxiety

♦ Extreme nervousness

Extreme nervousness is often a result of deep-seated fears that must be addressed in various ways, including with psychiatric help, but can be reduced on the surface by controlled deep breathing prior to performance.

- 41. Easy Seated Posture (or sit on a straight chair): Sit comfortably and quietly, spine straight, body relaxed, eyes closed
- *Anuloma Ujjāyī:* IN both nostrils/EX alternate nostrils (see chart 7.1; also chapter 3)

Chart 7.1

IN *U*	EX *l*	IN *U*	EX *r*	X
4	4	4	4	4
4	6	4	6	2
4	8	4	8	2
4	12	4	12	4
4	8	4	8	1
4	6	4	6	1
4	4	4	4	2

U (Ujjāyī) = throat (in this case, just both nostrils without sound to avoid drying the vocal folds); *l* = left nostril; *r* = right nostril

- 1. Balanced Standing Posture: Standing, do a shorter version of the practice in chart 7.1 (see chart 7.2)

Chart 7.2

IN U	EX l	IN U	EX r	X
4	4	4	4	2
4	6	4	6	1
4	8	4	8	1
4	12	4	12	1
4	8	4	8	1
4	6	4	6	1
4	4	4	4	2

· Do the seated breathing practice on the day of performance as often as you feel nervous, and the standing part during the last few minutes before performance.

♦♦ Mental blocks from early experiences

Early negative experiences associated with singing (or sometimes just with joyful behavior, such as a naturally loud speaking voice) can be very difficult to overcome. Basically, they must be identified, brought into consciousness, felt, accepted for what they really were, and forgiven in order to let them disappear. A meditation practice that allows feelings and thoughts to come to the surface of a quiet mind for acceptance and healing is one path to letting these blocks go. Sometimes the process is referred to as "untying knots" in the psyche. If what arises is too overwhelming, sitting with a trusted person who understands the practice is recommended.

· 41. Easy Seated Posture (or sit on a straight chair)
· Sitting with a straight spine, body relaxed, eyes closed, begin to be aware of your breathing
· Focus first on breathing at the belly—the rise and fall of the belly on IN and EX—for a few breaths
· Now bring your awareness to the sensations of the breath flowing inside the nostrils—cool and dry coming in, warm and moist going out
· Lengthen the breath to IN6/EX6 for 6–12 breaths until the mind is quiet
· Continuing your focus on the breath, allow the breath to assume its natural tides

- As thoughts or feelings arise, name each one twice ("thinking, thinking," "anger, anger," "planning, planning," "resisting, resisting," etc.) and gently return awareness to the breath
- When—or if—a feeling or memory connected to singing arises, simply allow it to be in your consciousness without judgment or resistance until it disappears of its own accord; accept its presence and the feeling it brings
- As thoughts and feelings arise and disappear in the context of the breath and silence, their impermanence becomes evident
- When you are ready to end your sit, return to IN6/EX6 for 6–12 breaths before rising

This type of meditation practiced daily begins to unload the psyche of its deep seated but unnecessary baggage. Some things may come up many times before they can finally be let go. Some issues that arise may need counseling help to resolve.

♦♦ Loss of breath capacity

Performance anxiety frequently manifests in severe breathlessness. This symptom can be alleviated by training the breath in a daily *prāṇāyāma* practice and by the use of a breathing practice prior to performance. The key is to develop a daily practice that emphasizes the deepening of the IN and the lengthening of the EX in various techniques.

- 41. Easy Seated Posture (or sit on a straight chair)
- First, find your present breath threshold (see chapter 3) that you can sustain comfortably for 12 breaths
- Using your comfortable threshold as a starting point, begin to work on lengthening your breath with a Ratio practice (see chapter 3) that lengthens the duration of one breath to at least 8:8:8:8
- Work up to this goal over several weeks or months
- This kind of daily practice will bring your breathing under conscious control as well as greatly strengthen the entire breathing mechanism
- Develop a short practice that you can use immediately before performance; for example, 4:4:8:4, an easy pattern that lengthens the exhale and calms the nervous system

◆ Loss of energy

Some singers experience a drop in energy just when they should have extra adrenaline for immediate performance.

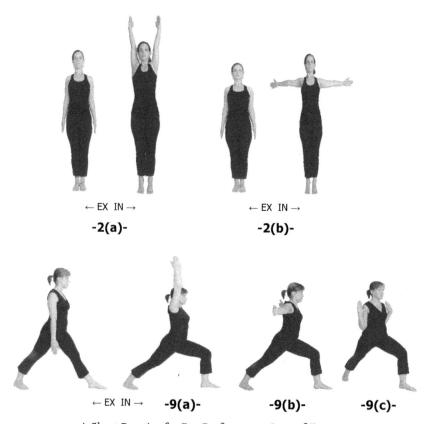

← EX IN →   ← EX IN →
-2(a)-   -2(b)-

← EX IN →   -9(a)-   -9(b)-   -9(c)-

FIGURE 11.24   A Short Practice for Pre-Performance Loss of Energy

· A short *Viloma Ujjāyī* breathing practice (see chapter 3) is energizing
· Follow the breathing practice with one or two postures that use arm raises coordinated with the breath to increase circulation and energy
   · 2. Mountain (a) and (b)
      · IN4/EX4 or IN2/EX4 x 4
      · Can also use a Ratio: 4:4:4:1; suspension after IN is energizing
   · 9. Warrior with arm variations
      · IN4/EX4 or IN2/EX4 x 6 (2 each arm variation), each side
      · Can also use a Ratio as above

Memory difficulties

If a singer is well prepared, memory blocks are usually due to nervousness or fear based on a negative past experience. The mind needs to be relaxed to function at its best. A daily practice of concentration/meditation techniques that includes both mental practice of music to be sung and some visualization of oneself giving a relaxed, flawless performance will condition the nervous system to function smoothly rather than interfere.

- 41. Easy Seated Posture: sitting with a straight spine, body relaxed, eyes closed
- Bring your awareness to the sensations of breath flowing inside the nostrils
- Lengthen the breath to IN6/EX6 x12 without losing your focus
- When your mind is quieter, visualize yourself giving a relaxed, flawless performance; feel the ease and joy of your singing in your whole body
- Now mentally sing through a song or aria with the same sense of ease and joy
- If words escape you, mentally embody the word or phrase that you missed and repeat it several times with a sense of ease
- Repeat the practice for each song or aria to be sung

Anxiety, Anger, and Depression

The states of anxiety, anger, and depression are emotional states that can range from normal responses to external stimuli to more neurotic tendencies that are psychologically based, to severe states based in abnormal biochemistry. The level of severity will indicate what kind of treatment is appropriate. Those states that are biochemical in origin must be treated medically, while those that are psychological in origin are best treated psychiatrically. In both cases, the goal is a change from extreme emotional reaction, thought, and behavior to a more balanced use of one's energies. This sometimes requires a 180-degree change of perception, thought, and subsequent behavior.

Finding balance and clarity is one of the great goals of the practice of yoga. For this reason, a well-designed yoga practice to fit the needs of the individual can be a valuable complement to whatever medical or psychiatric treatment is applied to the unbalanced emotional state. For the normal to moderate intermittent unbalanced emotional states, a committed yoga practice that includes physical, mental, and meditative elements will often not only alleviate the symptoms but can, over time, help to root out the habitual causes of imbalance.

Singers, because of the constant public exposure of their inmost selves in their singing, are particularly vulnerable to states of anxiety and sometimes depression as direct results of stress. If there is also an element of underlying unresolved imbalance, such as anger, the vulnerability is increased. For this reason, a daily healthful practice such as yoga that addresses body, mind, and spirit is necessary to retain the balance, clarity, and freedom to pursue the art of singing.

A few guidelines may help the reader to assess his or her own emotional state. The balanced emotional state, called *sattvic* in yoga philosophy, is characterized by emotions and attitudes that include "appreciation, awe, bliss, compassion, contentment, courage, forgiveness, friendliness, goodness, happiness, honesty, joy, kindness, love, patience, peace, serenity, stability, tenderness, tolerance, and wonder."[1] These emotions and attitudes are recognized by modern scientific research as factors that strengthen the immune system.

Anxiety and anger are called *rajasic* states of energy in yoga philosophy and are extremes of the same energy that fuels activity and creativity. The emotions and attitudes associated with anxiety include "agitation, apprehension, compulsiveness, concern, dread, edginess, fear, horror, insecurity, nervousness, obsessiveness, panic, paranoia, phobia, surprise, terror, uneasiness, wariness, and worry."[2] The emotions and attitudes associated with anger include "animosity, annoyance, aversion, criticism, cruelty, enmity, hostility, hatred, impatience, indignation, irritation, rage, resentment, violence, and wrath."[3]

Both strong anxiety and anger trigger the fight-or-flight response, which can produce such symptoms as "sweating, accelerated heartbeat, tightness in the belly, muscle tension, shakiness of the limbs, inability to be still or to concentrate, shortness of breath, and insomnia."[4] These emotional and physical states are recognized in scientific research to contribute to stress-related illnesses and to depress the immune system.

Depression is an extreme form of the *tamasic* quality of energy that governs stability but becomes inertia when it is out of balance. Emotions and attitudes associated with depression include "complacency, dejection, despair, disappointment, emptiness, gloom, grief, hopelessness, loneliness, melancholy, sadness, sorrow, self-pity, and shame."[5] The active and creative energy necessary to joyful and productive living is absent, and this lack affects negatively the body's ability to recover from illness. When clinical (biochemical) in nature, depression can become life threatening and must be medically treated.

As with anxiety and anger, depression requires some way to change underlying conditions to restore balance. There are currently ongoing studies that are beginning to indicate the beneficial effects of the practice of yoga on depression and even post-traumatic stress disorder (PTSD). The elements of yoga not only condition body and mind but also provide avenues to deeper insight into the psyche and personality, as well as techniques to effect change of perception, thought, and behavior.

The field of Yoga Therapy is currently in its formative stage, and there are numerous teachers who are also therapists. A leading figure in this emerging field is Gary Kraftsow, whose book *Yoga for Wellness* was one of the first of its kind. Chapter 5 of Kraftsow's book, "Emotional Health," gives much basic information on anxiety and depression, including case studies and practices designed for these individuals. They are excellent examples of how yoga can be helpful for these conditions.

Short Practices for Specific Situations

Energy States

♦ Low energy

These practices are good if you are tired in the morning or other times during the day; use IN4/EX4 for all postures

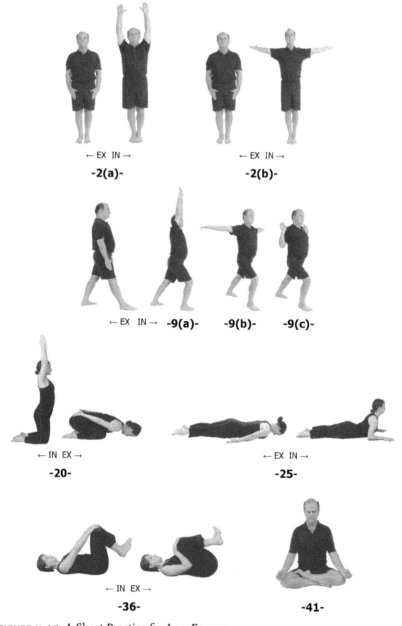

FIGURE 11.25 A Short Practice for Low Energy

In general, backward bending postures and breathing practices that emphasize inhalation are energizing. For example, if you are lethargic when you awaken in the morning (or after a nap or at other times during the day), a brief physical sequence plus a short energizing breathing practice will help get you moving.

- 2. Mountain (a) (b): x4 each; to stretch, breathe, and bring circulation to the whole body
- 9. Warrior: x6 each side with arm variations; to energize spine and legs
- 20. Kneeling Forward Bend: x4; transition to floor and between backward bends
- 25. Cobra: x4; to work the spinal muscles strongly
- 36. Supine Forward Bend: x4; compensation for backward bending
- 41. Easy Seated Posture: *Viloma Ujjāyī* (see chapter 3)

♦ Extreme morning tiredness

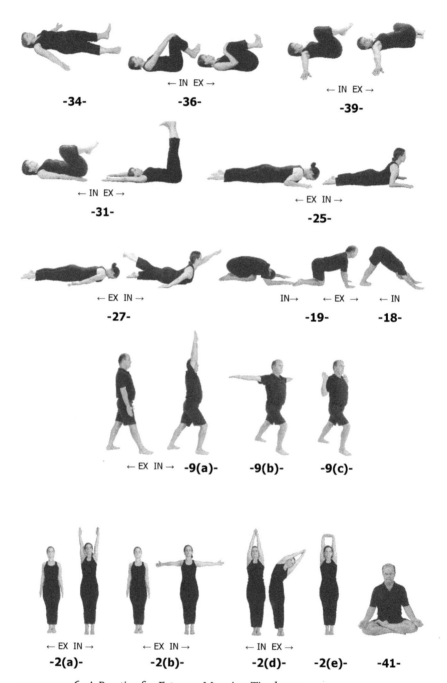

FIGURE II.26 A Practice for Extreme Morning Tiredness

If you are extremely tired in the morning, a more gradual awakening may be better. Use IN4/EX4

- 34. Corpse: take stock of how your body feels
- 36. Supine Forward Bend: x4; gently stretch the lower back
- 39. Supine Abdominal Twist (with knees bent): x4 each side; gently wake up the spine
- 31. Upward Feet Posture: x2; stretch legs and arms
- 25. Cobra: x4; activate the upper back muscles
- 27. Half Locust: x2 alternate sides; coordinate opposite sides of the body
- 19. Ruddy Goose: x4; compensation for backward bending
- 18. Downward Facing Dog: stay 4 breaths; stretch backs of legs and bring circulation to head in semi-inverted position
- 9. Warrior: x6 each side with arm variations; loosen the shoulders, open the chest, activate the legs, and deepen the breath
- 2. Mountain with arm and heel raises: (a), (b), (d), (e); a full wakeup
- 41. Easy Seated Posture: *Viloma Ujjāyī* (see chapter 3)

♦ Excessive energy

This practice is helpful if you are wired at bedtime or other times during the day; use IN4/EX4

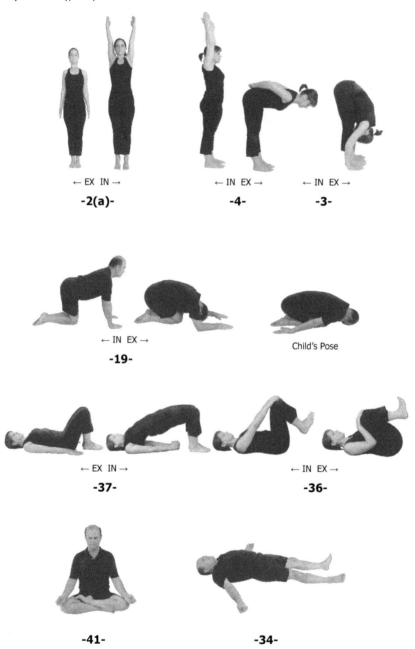

FIGURE 11.27 A Short Practice for Excessive Energy

In general, forward bending postures and breathing practices that emphasize exhalation are calming. For example, if you are "'wired" at bedtime, a short physical sequence plus a longer calming breathing practice will help to lower your level of energy.

- 2. Mountain: (a) x4; to use some excess energy
- 4.3. Standing Forward Bend: halfway x2; full bend, stay 4 breaths; to emphasize exhalation and to close the front of the body
- 19. Ruddy Goose: x4; rest in Child's Pose for a few breaths to relax
- 37. Bridge: x4; to compensate for forward bending
- 36. Supine Forward Bend: x4; to emphasize exhalation and close the front of the body
- 41. Easy Seated Posture: *Anuloma Ujjāyī* (see chapter 3)
- 34. Corpse: Continue focus on the breath; feel as if your whole body is breathing

If you are still tense and anxious, finish with a deep relaxation technique. Two are suggested below. If you are extremely tense, use both techniques in sequence.

- Tense and relax muscles progressively (see chapter 6)
- 31 or 61 Points Deep Relaxation (see chapter 6)

Restless mind

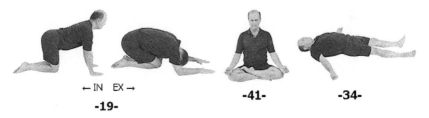

← IN EX →

-19-

-41-

-34-

FIGURE 11.28 A Short Practice for Restless Mind

Sometimes the mind simply will not slow down enough to focus on the task at hand or to sleep. This is the time to do a longer breathing practice followed by a concentration or meditation practice. Begin with a simple forward bend to stretch the back and emphasize exhalation. Then take a comfortable seated position and begin to focus on your breathing.

- 19. Ruddy Goose: x4–6
- 41. Easy Seated Posture: Sit with a straight spine, body relaxed, eyes closed
- Bring your awareness to the sensations of the breath flowing inside the nostrils
- Lengthen your breath to IN6/EX6; x12 without losing your focus
- You may wish to do a short *Nādi Śodhna* practice at this point (see chapter 3) using a 1:1:1:1 ratio, working up to 6:6:6:6 or 8:8:8:8, returning gradually to IN6/EX6 breath
- Begin mentally to say or hear the syllables "So-hum"—"So" on the IN and "Hum" on the EX; make each mental vowel sound as long as the breath (6 seconds), letting your awareness merge with the sound; be totally present in the inner sound
- As mental distractions arise, notice what each one is and gently return to "So-hum"
- Continue until your mind becomes quieter and you feel a sense of equilibrium in mind and body
- 34. Corpse: Rest for two or three minutes—or go directly to sleep

Travel and Performance

♦ After travel

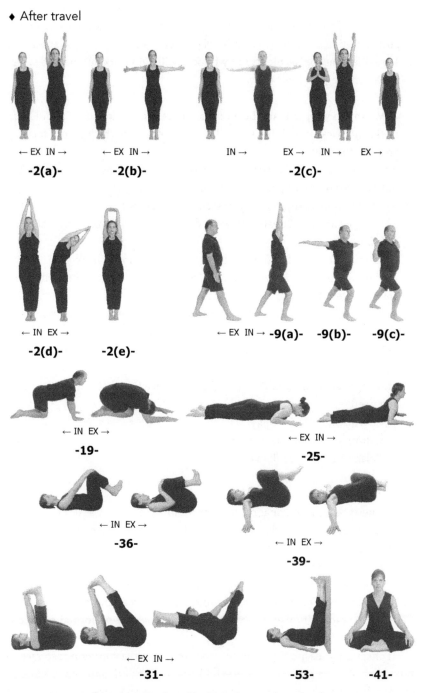

FIGURE II.29 A Short Practice for After Travel

For the working singer, travel is a constant fact of life. Most travel is tiring, and air travel has numerous hazards for the singer: dehydration, cramped sitting, danger of airborne illness, and the general tension of air travel, including airport conditions. Upon arrival at hotel or home, a short period of stretching and breathing, as well as plenty of hydration, will help work out the kinks. Use IN4/EX4 in the postures below.

- 2. Mountain with arm and heel raises, full sequence: to loosen shoulders, neck, and back, stretch the spine, bring circulation to the legs and feet, and breathe fully
- 9. Warrior: x6 each side with arm variations; to open the chest and work the muscles of the upper back and legs
- 19. Ruddy Goose: x6; to gently stretch the lower back
- 25. Cobra: x4; stay 2 breaths; to work the back muscles and invigorate the spine
- 36. Supine Forward Bend: x6 to gently stretch the lower back
- 39. Supine Abdominal Twist: x4 each side; stay 2–4 breaths; to rotate the spine, loosen the neck, and stretch the shoulders
- 31. Supine Big Toe Holding with Spread Legs: close legs slowly x2–4; to stretch the legs and work the inner thigh muscles
- 53. Legs Up the Wall: stay 5–15 minutes to relax and increase circulation to legs
- 41. Easy Seated Posture: Do a breathing practice for whatever energy state you need
  - Energizing: *Viloma Ujjāyī*
  - Calming: *Anuloma Ujjāyī*
  - Balancing: *Nādi Śodhana*

Before performance

Most singers have a personal routine for performance days, and the needs of each person are different depending on individual temperament. Some singers have excess energy and/or nervous tension; some have a low energy level until just before performance time. For those who have developed a yoga practice, there are many choices of physical and mental practices to fine-tune for the performance. For most singers, some form of breathing practice is helpful. Which practice to use depends on the habitual pre-performance breath patterns of the individual.

If chest muscles are tight and breath seems short (a common response to the stress of anticipation), do a breathing practice that lengthens the breath cycle with emphasis on a long exhalation to calm the nervous system (*Anuloma*

Ujjāyī or a simple ratio) followed by emphasis on inhalation to open the chest. If energy seems low, do a short breathing practice that builds energy (*Viloma Ujjāyī* or a simple ratio). If you feel distracted or off center, do an alternate nostril practice (before makeup, of course) for balancing energy (*Nādi Śodhana*). If your mind is racing, do a simple IN6/EX6 "So-hum" concentration practice to slow down and focus.

After performance

After the performance and celebrations are over, it is often difficult to wind down for sleep, especially if much food has been consumed. If there are a few minutes of private time between the end of the performance and the after-performance activities, while changing from costume into street clothes, for example, a few gentle forward bends and a short breathing practice (such as *Anuloma Ujjāyī*) that emphasizes exhalation would begin the process of winding down. It is not advisable, however, to do forward bends after eating. If falling asleep is a problem, a simple concentration practice (such as focusing on the breath or using a mantra such as "So-hum") will help to quiet the mind.

Weight Issues

Our society encourages mindless eating. We eat on the run, in noisy environments, while multitasking at work, in front of the computer, watching television, driving the car. We eat in social situations, as reward, for comfort, from boredom. We eat too late at night or not at all in the morning. We eat too much or not enough, too often or not often enough. The body almost never has the chance to do its work of digestion in a normal and regular cycle without interference. Rarely do we sit down in a quiet environment and truly pay attention to the wonderful experience of eating a meal in which we are keenly aware of the color, flavor, texture, and motions of each bite. It is an experience with which most of us are almost totally unacquainted.

Many singers struggle with weight issues. For some, these issues were created early in life, either from family eating patterns or as a coping mechanism for dealing with stress. For others the main issue is the avoidance of weight gain in a profession that often skews the normal and healthy eating cycle into a delicious hazard of late-night, post-performance parties and after-rehearsal meals. These eating opportunities usually occur in a convivial social situation in which attention is on conversation while eating, and who knows what, let alone how much, was just ingested? They are usually followed by falling into bed for a good night's sleep, barring indigestion. This scenario is the perfect setup for the dreaded weight gain, as well as one of the singer's greatest enemies, acid reflux.

The two types of issues described above generally require somewhat different approaches to a solution, but both rest squarely on the individual's relationship to his or her own body and on the relationship between the individual's psyche and food itself. The act of eating has many faces, and finding the right one for oneself is not easy if the process has become unhealthy. The great American diet industry makes billions of dollars each year offering various types of solutions to the issue of too many pounds of fat weighing us down. Most of the commercial approaches emphasize physical appearance as the goal while medically prescribed approaches emphasize the benefits to health. In general, the health benefit approaches are more realistic and safer to pursue. Almost all, however, are based on some sort of deprivation—or perceived deprivation—of one of our favorite daily activities: eating the foods we love. This is especially difficult for singers, as singing and eating delicious food go so well together.

This brings us to the investigation of the two relationships set forth above: the singer's relationship to his or her own body, and the relationship between the singer's psyche and food itself. It seems to be a truism that many singers do not have a good relationship with their own bodies. Some actively dislike their bodies at some level, and some are simply unaware of the intimate connection between singing and the body. Either of these non-relationships can be detrimental to singing when one considers that the singing instrument is the whole body itself and not the voice alone.

One of the major goals of the practice of yoga is to become intimately acquainted with one's body in positive ways. The physical postures and breathing practices offer many avenues to this knowledge and, along the way, condition and refine the body for whatever purpose is desired. Beyond working directly with the body and breath, yoga enters the field of the mind to investigate its contents; its stream of consciousness; its conditioned views, reactions, and responses; and the relationships it creates with the body and the senses. Since the mind is the coordinator of the senses, organizing and interpreting the incoming sensory information, it is reasonable to say that the mind itself is where the work must be done when sensory issues—such as overeating— get out of balance. Here is where perceptions—such as deprivation—can be investigated, understood, and reformed.

The lack of a loving connection between body and psyche often has its roots in early experiences. If the singer who carries excessive weight that will block opportunities to sing has a body type formed in childhood, some deep investigation of the psychic connection to food will probably be necessary before embarking on a solution. Once identified, the mental and emotional connections can become a part of a daily practice in "untying the knots" that bind one to unhealthy habits. This process occurs in the practice of meditation (see practices for similar issues in "Mental blocks from early experiences"). Ultimately, when one's body is accepted for the marvelous creation that it is, it is time to turn attention to the relationship between the psyche and food or, more precisely, the act of eating.

The act of eating is often mindless; that is, we are not fully aware of the process, especially if eating accompanies another activity. Some of these other activities, mentioned at the beginning of this discussion, are common to all of us at one time or another. Our society encourages us to eat more and more as serving portions become larger and larger, and eating out in the company of friends becomes more and more common. Indeed, almost every social interaction involves food. What happens to the energy in all this food we consume? What does it do for—or to—our bodies, our minds? These are questions worth asking in the context of discovering what it means to eat mindfully.

Eating mindfully can relate to many different levels of human activity, but the most immediate level for the purposes of this discussion is the direct relationship between one's awareness and the act of eating. The simplest definition of being present in the present moment is to know what one is doing while one is doing it. How often, for example, do you misplace something important because at the moment you put that something down your mind was busy elsewhere? It happens all the time. We tend to live mentally in the next time frame, or in the previous one. The act of eating often takes place while we are mentally or physically doing something else. At best this cancels the enjoyment of eating; at worst it often leads to overeating.

What does it mean to eat mindfully, and how does one do it? Stephen Levine devotes thirty pages of his book *Guided Meditations, Explorations and Healings* to this topic.[6] Personally acquainted with extreme addiction as a young man, Levine has great insight into how desire and the drive to satisfy desire rule our lives until and unless we do the work of taking that power away from our senses and giving it to our consciousness. The titles of some of the sections give an overview of their content: "An Exploration of Eating"; "Taking a Single Bite Meditation"; "A Further Inquiry into Eating"; "The Fork Story"; "Eating Meditation—A Note about Technique"; "Eating Play: An Experiment in Consciousness." Two previous sections set up the context for this approach: "The Chain of Events" and "Itching Play: An Experiment in Consciousness."

For singers whose eating patterns approach addiction and who are serious about changing those patterns, reading and experimenting with the wisdom in these pages of Levine's book could be a turning point. Indeed, the insights and practices given would be valuable to anyone who wishes to make adjustments in attitude toward and relationship to food. The general approach is first to become conscious of the chain of events that leads from desire to the action taken to fulfill that desire: desire—intention—action. The focal point is intention, which is the only point at which we can stop unconsciously repeating old habits. Once this process is understood, the next step is to practice being in the moment of whatever we are doing—in this case, eating.

The practices of mindful eating given by Levine direct us to notice every single thing in succession about taking a single bite of food: sitting down, feeling the body in the chair, looking at the table setting, seeing the food on the plate, noticing color and shape, reaching for the fork, noticing how it feels in the hand, being aware of the muscular action of the arm and hand in putting food on the fork and lifting it to the mouth, smelling the aroma of the food, taking the food into the mouth, putting the fork down, appreciating the first burst of flavor, chewing, swallowing, noticing the desire for more. It is eating one bite of food in slow motion, noticing color, flavor, texture, the motions of hand, mouth, teeth, and throat. It is being completely present in each moment, moment to moment. It is noticing the workings of the mind in the chain of desire, intention, and action. Noticing all of this as it happens brings insight into the process and the ability to create a new vision of what it means to eat.

At first glance, the approach of eating mindfully each bite of an entire meal may seem overwhelming and impossible. Indeed, it is not a practice that can be undertaken under our everyday circumstances. It would need to be considered an experiment in a specific time set aside for the experience. For example, plan it for an hour when eating alone in a quiet environment without interruption is possible. Prepare a meal well balanced with respect to color, flavor, and texture, and eat it mindfully, one bite at a time (putting down the fork after each bite), noticing everything that Levine recommends in "Taking a Single Bite Meditation."[7] Doing this practice just one time will sow the seeds of a different attitude toward eating, even if the experience is exasperating. Doing the practice with one meal a day for three weeks will encourage a substantial mental shift in the relationship between psyche and the act of eating. From this basis, the practice can be used perhaps once a week just to keep everything on track.

Learning to appreciate fully what it means to eat mindfully will carry over in some measure to all other eating, and can also forge a pathway to mindfulness in other activities as well. Being aware in the moment is the precursor to being in balance in all things. Finding balance in eating leads to better health, more energy, easier movement, and a more loving relationship to the body, which, in turn, leads to a deeper relationship with the whole of life.

Losing or preventing the gain of excessive weight is scientifically a matter of how many calories come in as food and how many calories go out as energy each day. To lose pounds, the income must be less than the outgo; to maintain, the income and outgo must balance each other. The concept of "dieting" often ends up doing more harm than good because of the actual or subconscious feeling of deprivation. In reality, any food that is not actively harmful to the individual system is suitable for inclusion in one's daily meals. The question is how much and when? The important thing is to know and have a good relationship between the body and food. The key is mindful eating. Mindful eating tends to slow down the process, providing a satisfying eating experience and giving the stomach time to signal when it is full. This in turn leads to fewer calories consumed.

To return to the concept of developing mindfulness through the practice of meditation, almost everyone has a very favorite food, something that is craved and cannot be passed up when opportunity arises. Sometimes this favorite food, usually containing many calories and unlikely to be celery, becomes a daily item, perhaps associated with a specific activity such as practicing, rehearsing, studying, reading, watching television, or working at the computer. Perhaps the favorite food is seen as a reward for work done. An example is the ever present giant-size soft drink. The links between desire and gratification concerning this item become incredibly strong and form deep habits in the neural pathways of the brain. In chapter 4 of this book, a practice for "weakening and letting go of old thought habits" is applicable to the issue at hand. Based on information from brain-imaging research, this practice helps to weaken the emotional charge attached to a particular habit by weakening the neural connection associated with it in the brain.

Taking the giant-size soft drink as an example—or chocolate, or chips, or whatever is a strong habit—sit in a meditation position with eyes closed and, after focusing on the breath for a few minutes, allow the awareness to rest on a mental picture of the food object. Simply rest awareness on the object, without judgment or engagement, and notice how the mind is drawn into the cycle of desire. Then shift awareness to no focus at all, or to the breath. When the mind wanders toward the object, allow the awareness to rest again without judgment or engagement on the food object. Continue this oscillation between the food object and no focus or focus on the breath. After a few minutes, notice whether the mind remains a little calmer when awareness is on the food object. Making this a daily or twice daily practice for a period of days or weeks, notice whether the compulsion to indulge has weakened, whether it is possible to bypass the food at will.

This is one of the many ways that the practice of meditation develops mindfulness for a specific need. This simple practice can be used to help weaken any undesirable habit or to form a desirable habit. The practice can be done formally in a seated position at a specific time and place or informally at any time and place when a minute or two is available. Frequency of practice yields the best results.

In conclusion, the issue of too much weight for singers is a serious consideration, especially if a singer is well on the way to having a performing career. Most people who have tried different weight-loss diets know how ineffective they can be, and not necessarily because they are not reasonable approaches. The fault lies not in our diets but in our minds. Knowing how the mind works in the chain of desire-intention-action, and knowing that chain reaction can be interrupted and ultimately changed is the foundation of the solution to achieving and maintaining one's best weight.

Afterword

The principles, techniques, and practices set forth in this book are best learned in a class setting and practiced both in class and individually in a regular personal practice. For this reason, it is highly desirable to have ongoing yoga classes designed especially for singers as a part of the voice curriculum at the university level or in another venue. Those singers who are also voice teachers are the primary individuals to investigate the possibilities of implementing such classes. Voice teachers or other singers who also practice yoga, are the ideal individuals to consider teaching such classes. An overview of two semesters of yoga classes designed for singers is presented in the appendix.

With this in mind, the author offers workshops to acquaint voice teachers with the benefits of yoga to their students, as well as teacher training for those who are interested in teaching yoga classes for singers. A link to information about workshops and training can be found on the Companion Web site to this book.

For the Voice Teacher

Yoga for the Private Lesson

The private lesson is generally all too short to achieve a desired goal. There are so many facets of the art of singing that must come together into a single act that it is sometimes difficult to know how to proceed. If only there were a few simple tools to apply on the spot to the basic techniques that need to be developed, perhaps much time could be saved. For students and teachers who have no access to an appropriate yoga class, a few simple practices can be easily learned and used.

The following yoga practices are offered for just such situations. Each one is designed to be used in the private lesson for a specific purpose. Each can be done in a standing or sitting position, and each is simple enough to be used by teachers and students unacquainted with yoga.

♦ Posture and Alignment

- 9. Warrior: (c) IN4/EX4 x4 each side; stay 2–4 breaths last time; bent knee straight over ankle, heels firmly on floor, chest over thigh, pelvis back, hands in line with shoulders, shoulder blades pulled together and down, head pulled back in line with spine, chin strongly down

This posture greatly strengthens the muscles of the upper back and shoulders, lengthens the back of the neck (when head is moved back in line with the spine and chin lowered), works the muscles of inhalation, and strengthens the legs. The student should practice this posture twice a day for three months, or as long as it takes to develop the upper back strength to keep the chest up and open and the head back and shoulders down for good singing posture. The strong tucked chin position in the posture is for muscle training purposes and is not suggested for actual singing posture. Each singer will need a different degree of chin position correction, depending on overall posture.

Breathing Technique

Many beginning singers do not know the location and action of their breathing muscles. It is helpful to see a picture or drawing of these muscles but even more helpful to feel their action. A yoga breathing practice called *Krama* (segmented) is an excellent way to locate and feel the action of the breathing muscles. In this seated practice the breath is both inhaled and exhaled in segments with pauses in between.

- *Krama* Breathing Practice (Segmented Breathing; see chapter 3)
- Sit either on a straight chair with spine away from the back of the chair or cross legged on the floor
- Place the right hand on the chest and the left hand on the belly
- Locate the following points on the front of the body: pubic bone, navel, solar plexus, sternum
- Sit with a straight spine, relaxed shoulders, jaw, and tongue, eyes closed for concentration
- Depending on which breathing technique is taught in the studio, choose the appropriate type of inhalation
- ♦ Two-segment breath: using a 4-count IN/4-count EX, begin to inhale either from the sternum down, or from the belly up, whichever the teacher prefers
    - IN counts 1 and 2 from sternum to navel (or from pubic bone to navel) PAUSE (suspend the breath and stop motion)
    - IN 3 and 4 from navel to pubic bone (or from navel to sternum) PAUSE
    - EX 1 and 2 from pubic bone to navel PAUSE
    - EX 3 and 4 from navel to sternum PAUSE
    - Repeat several times, noticing which muscles are engaged and what direction they are moving (down and out, or up and in)
- ♦♦ Three-segment breath: using a 6-count IN/6-count EX, repeat the above exercise in three segments
    - IN counts 1 and 2 from sternum to solar plexus (or from pubic bone to navel) PAUSE
    - IN 3 and 4 from solar plexus to navel (or from navel to solar plexus) PAUSE
    - IN 5 and 6 from navel to pubic bone (or from solar plexus to sternum) PAUSE
    - EX 1 and 2 from pubic bone to navel PAUSE
    - EX 3 and 4 from navel to solar plexus PAUSE

- EX 5 and 6 from solar plexus to sternum PAUSE
- Repeat several times, noticing which muscles are engaged and what direction they are moving

This practice not only shows the singer where the breathing muscles are and how they move, but also strengthens the musculature of the entire breathing mechanism and develops attention to the breath and concentration on the task at hand. Repeated daily, this short practice will help the singer become fully aware of the breathing mechanism and process.

Breath Control

Breath control is a separate function from breathing technique but depends upon a solid breathing technique for its development. In general, singers are most concerned about the length of their breath in a sung phrase and, secondarily, about the ability to take in enough air quickly for the next phrase when a longer inhalation is impossible. Given the fact that in performance, breath issues are often complicated by the impact of nervousness on the breath, the consistent daily practice of yoga breathing exercises has a double result: a longer breath span for singing *and* the ability to use the breath to calm the nervous system. The following two breathing practices are designed to increase breath capacity, gain control over the relationship between inhalation and exhalation, and lengthen exhalation for the singing of long phrases. Both practices are done in a seated position.

♦ Breath Threshold (see chapter 3)
- Sit on a straight chair or cross-legged on the floor with a straight spine, relaxed shoulders, arms, jaw, and tongue, eyes closed
- Bring awareness to the sensations of breath flowing inside the nostrils
- Lengthen the IN and EX to 4 counts each x4
- Begin to lengthen the count to 6:6 x4; 8:8 x4; 10:10, 12:12 if comfortable, each x4
- When you have reached your maximum comfortable breath length, do 12 cycles; if 12 is too strenuous, revert to a shorter count
- Beginning at your comfortable length—your breath threshold—gradually increase the length by one or two counts at a time to develop a greater breath capacity; do this practice daily for a month

♦♦ Breath Ratio (see chapter 3)
- Sit on a straight chair or cross-legged on the floor with a straight spine, relaxed shoulders, arms, jaw, and tongue, eyes closed
- Bring awareness to the sensations of breath flowing inside the nostrils

- Lengthen the IN and the EX to 4 counts each x4 and do the practice shown in chart A.1

Chart A.1

IN	SF	EX	SE	X
4	o	4	o	4
4	2	4	o	2
4	4	4	o	2
4	2	4	2	2
4	o	4	4	2
4	2	4	4	2
4	4	4	4	4 (or 12)
4	o	4	o	4

IN = inhale; SF = suspend breath with lungs full; EX = exhale; SE = suspend breath with lungs empty; X = number of repetitions

When the 4:4:4:4 breath (16 seconds) is easy, increase to 6:6:6:6 and 8:8:8:8, building up each time with the pattern in the chart (that is, 6:3:6:3, 6:4:6:4, 6:6:6:6; 8:4:8:4, 8:6:8:6, 8:8:8:8, etc.).

When the overall breath is of sufficient length, begin to shorten the IN and SF and lengthen the EX and SE to create a relationship of Inhale to Exhale that is more like singing a series of phrases. Remember that the SE phase of the breath increases the length of the Exhalation capacity; for example, 4:2:8:4; 2:2:8:8; 1:2:8:8; 1:2:12:6; 1:2:16:4, and so on. The possibilities are as many as there are different phrase lengths in songs.

The student should practice ratio breathing exercises on a daily basis to lengthen the breath and strengthen the overall breathing mechanism. It is also possible to construct a ratio breathing practice to mirror the phrase structure of a particular song (see chapter 3).

Mental Focus

Sometimes students come to the voice lesson with a lot on their minds other than singing. In these cases, unless the lesson will be one of those "talk sessions" that seem to be needed from time to time, it is useful to have a short concentration practice to clear the mind and focus on the task at hand. This can be something as simple as having the student stand at the piano with closed eyes and focus on the sensations of the breath flowing inside the nostrils. When the focus is established, lengthen the breath to IN6/EX6 for a few breaths. Instruct the student to notice when distracting thoughts or feelings arise in the mind, notice what each one is, and gently return the focus to the breath.

After about a minute of this concentration, instruct the student to open the eyes, focus on a point in space several feet away and slightly down, shift the weight to one leg, and lift the other knee forward until the thigh is parallel to the floor. Maintain the visual focus and one-legged balance for two to four breaths. Arms may be at sides, hands on hips, or hands together at the chest or overhead. Repeat on the opposite side. This kind of balance posture develops concentration on a single point. Distraction will cause a loss of balance. After these two brief concentration exercises, the student should be more focused and ready to proceed with the lesson.

Yoga for Singers Classes: Lesson Plan Introductions and Outlines

The outline of lesson plans for two semesters of yoga classes for voice students, or for a series of yoga classes for singers in settings other than the university, is intended to help the teacher of such classes by providing a progressive overall structure and formats for individual classes. Voice teachers or other singers who also practice yoga and have some teacher training are the ideal teachers for such classes, as they would have knowledge and experience in both areas.

The material presented in this Appendix is an introduction to the concept of structured, progressive yoga classes for singers using the principles set forth in the main text. The principles and techniques for teaching these classes are best experienced and learned in a live class setting. For this reason, the class material is available in workshops. A short demonstration class can be viewed on the Companion Website. ⏵ For those voice teachers who are interested in teaching the classes, teacher training is also available from this author.

The class topics suggested here are designed to support the activities of student singers early in their training (or any other singers who have little or no acquaintance with the connections between yoga and singing)—for example, the freshman year at the college or university level. The progression of classes more or less parallels the usual order of beginning or intermediate voice lessons: posture and alignment, the breathing mechanism, and use of the breath in sound, as well as attention to the areas of mental focus, emotional openness, and relaxation. In addition, two first-semester classes offer approaches to unfamiliar vowel sounds in various languages and to memorizing music.

The class plans given here are introductions to and brief outlines of the material to be covered. Details and practices will be presented in workshops. The first semester classes can work in either a 50-minute period or a 75-minute period, depending on the time available in a given schedule. The shorter class period will be sufficient for the first series of classes. The second series of classes will need the 75-minute period for best results. One class per week is minimal to present the material. Two classes per week would allow time to reinforce the material before moving on to the next topic. Some topics may need more time than others and can be broken up into shorter units. Each teacher, depending on experience and training, will bring individual insights and ideas to this basic material. As always, the needs of the students will also help to shape the classes.

How the last class of a series is used depends on whether the class carries credit or is structured as an adjunct to the private lesson, much like performance classes. Some mechanism that encourages class attendance is desirable. The time of day of the class is also important. Yoga should be practiced on an empty stomach, so scheduling the class just before lunch or dinner is a good idea. Although most serious yoga practitioners tend to prefer a morning practice, scheduling a yoga class for college students before breakfast is almost guaranteed to fail.

It is important to convey to the students that yoga, like music, is a practice. It is something to incorporate into daily life, just as the practice of one's art is a daily practice. The great difference is that the practice of yoga serves the needs of the singer and may be different each day—shorter or longer, easy or more intense, made up of different components—whereas the practice of music requires the singer to serve the music. The practice of yoga enables the singer to serve the music better on almost every level.

First Semester
Fourteen Classes

Class 1
Introduction to Yoga for Singing

I. What Is Yoga?
(In some areas of the United States, it may be necessary to say what yoga is *not*, because of the lack of knowledge and the religious temperament of the population. In any case, it is always good practice to present yoga in the context of the mind-set of the students in the class.)
- Yoga is not
  - a religion; is not based on a set of beliefs; has no theology
  - a physical fitness exercise program
  - a competitive sport
- Yoga is
  - a tool for change—physical, mental, attitudinal, behavioral
  - an experiential system of practices that benefits every facet of the person—body, breath, mind, emotions, soul—and influences behavior
  - The word "yoga"
    - From the Indo-European root word "yuj" meaning "union," "to unite," "to yoke"
    - Refers to the uniting of two or more things

II. The Connections between Yoga and Singing
(see chapter 1: Yoga and Singing: The Connections)

III. Class Format

Although each class will have a specific focus on a yoga practice (or practices) that relates directly to some element of singing, all classes will contain the full range of a complete practice in some form. This will reinforce the value of all the areas of practice through class repetition.

The elements of yoga that form a complete practice are

- *Āsana* (physical postures) with breath and sound adaptations
- *Prāṇāyāma* (breathing practices) with Humming (exhalation applied to vocal sound)
- Concentration techniques
- Meditation techniques
- Deep relaxation techniques
- Each practice will be linked to a corresponding element of singing—but with no actual singing

IV. A Word about Practice

The most basic definition of "to practice" is "to repeat the lesson." The development of the body, breath, and mind, and the opening of the heart in yoga require repetition, just as the development of the voice and of musical skills requires repetition. With this in mind, it is important to make the connection between a daily yoga practice and progress in the elements of singing addressed by the various yoga practices. The more the student can see that yoga and singing are natural partners, the easier it will be to develop a consistent yoga practice that complements the daily practice of singing.

The easiest way to begin to develop a daily yoga practice is to repeat the contents of the class lesson during the week or days before the next class. One need not do all of the lesson at once, but practicing all the elements of the class at least twice before the next class will give the student an introduction to the skills upon which the next lesson will build.

V. An Abbreviated Sample Class (about 20 minutes)

- *Āsana* (Physical Postures) using IN4/EX4
    - 2. Mountain with arm and heel raises: (a) and (b) x4 each; (c) x2; (d) x2; (e) stay 3 breaths
    - 3. Standing Forward Bend: halfway x3; full bend, stay 2–4 breaths
    - 9. Warrior: x6 each side with arm variations; stay 2–4 breaths last time
    - 19. Ruddy Goose: x4
- *Prāṇāyāma* (Breathing Practices)
    - 41. Easy Seated Posture
    - Explore breath capacity (see chapter 3)
    - Hum "My Country, 'Tis of Thee" as far as possible on one breath (use a very light *pp* hum felt high on the bridge of the nose) to establish a benchmark of present breath length
- Concentration: "Yoga is the control of thought waves in the mind." (*Yoga Sutras of Patanjali*, Sutra I.2, Isherwood trans.)

- A practice of noticing and letting go of unwanted thoughts and feelings—the initial step in learning to control the "thought waves" in the mind
- Sitting with straight spine, head a little back and chin a little down, relaxed body, eyes closed, establish a smooth flowing 6IN/EX6 breath
- Focus on the sensations of the breath flowing inside the nostrils
- When thoughts or feelings arise and your attention wanders, notice where your attention went, and return awareness to the sensations of the breath in the nostrils
  - Relaxation: "Through relaxation we restore a sense of inner harmony"[1]
    - Lie on the back with straight spine, legs slightly apart, arms resting a little away from the body, palms up, eyes closed (*Śavāsana*)
    - Relax the forehead muscle, the eye muscles, the jaw and tongue, the thumbs, and the big toes
    - Allow your whole body to feel as if it is melting into the floor
    - Gently bring awareness back to your breathing; feel your whole body breathe, completely relaxed—body, breath, and mind
    - When you are ready, taking all the time you need, bring your awareness back to the room, move your hands and feet, open your eyes, stretch if needed, and return to sitting
  - Review succinctly how each practice above relates directly to singing
  - Q and A for any questions students might have

Class 2
Posture and Alignment

Chapter 2 contains information on the physical postures that relate to the various areas of the muscles of singing. Part II contains specific sequences for each area for the student. This class will focus on an *āsana* sequence that includes a few postures from each area in a progression that makes an effective overall sequence.

Bandhas (see chapter 3) are muscular contractions sometimes called "locks" that strengthen a particular set of muscles as well as having other beneficial effects. Of the three primary *bandhas*, the first two (*Jālandhara*, or chin lock, and *Uddīyāna*, or abdominal lock) are important for posture and alignment. The second, *Uddīyāna*, is also extremely important for breathing. The third (*Mūla*, or root lock) is also important for posture and breathing but will be introduced later.

The practice of *Jālandhara bandha* with certain postures brings the head into alignment with the spine, stretching the back of the neck and preventing the chin from jutting forward. This movement is taken after inhalation and kept throughout the practice of the posture. It need not be done to an extreme degree and will probably be different in degree with each individual's needs.

The practice of *Uddīyāna bandha* is a natural part of exhalation as well as functioning to stabilize the lower back in many postures. In its full form, it is taken after exhalation and kept for a predetermined length of time during the "Stay" part of the posture, greatly strengthening the abdominal muscles. This *bandha* comes into play gradually over the span of a long exhalation.

  I. *Āsana*: The Postural Muscles of Singing + Two *Bandhas*
 II. *Prānāyāma*: A Simple Breath Lengthening Practice
III. Concentration
IV. Relaxation

Class 3
The Breathing Mechanism

There are many wonderful materials available that show the breathing mechanism in great detail. Once the parts of the mechanism are identified in an illustration and then located in the singer's own body, it is time for development. The complexities of the act of singing often make it difficult to focus on just one aspect of the process while engaged in actual singing. For this reason, the breathing practices of yoga are of great help in developing the musculature of the breathing mechanism. This class will locate, explore, and begin to work with the mechanism that is the very foundation of the art of singing.

  I. *Āsana*: A Short Sequence
 II. *Prānāyāma*: Development of the Mechanism
III. Concentration
IV. Relaxation

Class 4
Breath in Movement

The use of various metrical breathing patterns in physical postures accomplishes several things. It strengthens the body as a whole by increasing the work being done and develops smooth muscular control in movement. It strengthens the breathing mechanism itself and expands and deepens breath control, especially if constructed to apply to lengthening exhalation. It trains attention in the present moment and enhances stability of the pulse in musical meter.

  I. Breath Adaptations in *Āsana*: Working with Breath Patterns
 II. *Prānāyāma*
III. Concentration
IV. Relaxation

Class 5
Prānāyāma and Humming I

The word *Prānāyāma* is a compound word in Sanskrit, *Prānā*, meaning the life force, human energy, often expressed as breath and *āyāma*, meaning expansion or control of; thus *Prānāyāma* is the expansion and control of the life force as breath. The term also refers to the various practices that lengthen and strengthen the breath in general. These practices applied to the art of singing are of incalculable value to the developing singer.

Prānāyāma work in classical yoga is preceded by *āsana* in which the breathing patterns prepare the breath for seated breathing practices. A short *āsana* sequence is sufficient to prepare the breath but not so long as to tire the body.

  I. *Āsana* with Breath Adaptations to Prepare for *Prānāyāma*
 II. *Prānāyāma*
III. Humming
IV. Concentration: Use of "So-hum"
 V. Relaxation

Class 6
Prānāyāma and Humming II

We begin this class with the same *āsana* sequence as that of Class 5 as an ongoing practice for postural development and strengthening the breathing mechanism through breath adaptations in the postures. New material includes two *prānāyāma* techniques and extended humming exercises.

  I. *Āsana* with Breath Adaptations to Prepare for *Prānāyāma*
 II. *Prānāyāma*
III. Humming
IV. Concentration
 V. Relaxation

Class 7
Sound in Āsana

At birth the first two things that happen are an inhalation and a sound. From that moment on, we are sound-producing beings. Sound has many properties. It is communication; it carries meaning, both cognitive and symbolic; it trains attention, carries energy, creates circulation, and intensifies the effects of an activity. Sound as music directly affects the nervous system; can change activity, mental state, and emotional mood; and can elevate or degrade the soul and spirit. All these properties of sound come into play in chanting and singing. The singer, more than anyone else, knows, embodies, and wields the power of all these aspects of sound.

The use of sound in *āsana* serves several functions. At the most basic level, the use of Italian vowel sounds as a chanting device lengthens the exhale as tone, helps to learn correct vowel sounds (especially those pure vowel sounds [e] and [o] that are diphthongs in English), helps to produce clear resonance in long tones, and serves as a focus of attention for movement. The *āsana* section of this class introduces the use of humming and of the seven Italian vowel sounds combined with movement.

   I. *Āsana* with Humming and Seven Italian Vowel Sounds
  II. *Prāṇāyāma*
 III. Humming
 IV. Concentration
  V. Relaxation

Class 8
Concentration Techniques

The waking mind is in constant motion. It is always busy—organizing and interpreting information from the senses, receiving emotional information, retrieving memories, judging the present, planning the future, reacting to external stimuli, and simply thinking about all sorts of things. Some of this activity is vital to our safety and well-being. Much of it is useless, distracting us from the present moment, arising uninvited to prevent us from seeing things as they really are. In this way, the mind is in control. Book 1, Verse 2, of the classic yoga text, *Yoga Sutras,* defines yoga as "the control of thought waves in the mind." This is far more difficult than the most advanced physical posture or breathing practice.

Gaining control over one's own mind involves the ability to focus on a single point for an extended period of time, allowing each mental distraction to arise and pass away of its own accord, merely noticing what the distraction is and returning attention to the single focus. This ability is cultivated through regular practice, just as singing well is cultivated through regular practice. Gradually the flood of distractions diminishes, and the immense quiet of the mind is experienced in brief moments. In these moments, one gets a flash of clarity, inner knowing (intuition) unclouded by previous experience. The one-pointed mind is a powerful tool in almost any situation.

Concentration is a seated practice usually preceded by *prāṇāyāma* and often followed by meditation. This means that one must be comfortable in a motionless seated posture that keeps the spine erect and the shoulders and arms relaxed for up to twenty or thirty minutes at one sitting. In accordance, the *āsana* practice for this class will focus on those postures that prepare the body to sit with as little discomfort as possible. It is useful to know that *āsana* prepares the body for *prāṇāyāma*, *prāṇāyāma* prepares the breath for concentration, and concentration prepares the mind for meditation.

   I. *Āsana:* A Sequence for Sitting Comfortably
  II. *Prāṇāyāma*
 III. Concentration
 IV. Relaxation

Class 9
Meditation Practices

Our personalities, perceptions, thoughts, emotions, and behaviors develop as a result of the conditioning given to or imposed upon us from childhood. Some of our conditioning serves us well and some does not. Some conditioning grounds us in our most fundamental values and some cripples us for life if we do not make the effort to escape it. Change is always possible because change is the nature of all life. What is needed is an opening through which we can see a different way to be.

In the context of classical yoga, the practice of meditation is such an opening. As referenced in chapter 5, the practice of meditation influences the personality just as the practices of *āsana* and *prāṇāyāma* influence the body and energy. Meditation is the state of mind that appears when a prolonged period of concentration has brought the mind to stillness. This stillness often first appears as an instant of recognition that the mind is quiet. Longer periods of mental silence usually come only with consistent practice over a long period of time.

No one can say what "should happen" in meditation. What appears, or does not appear, is unique to each individual and ultimately leads inward toward the heart. The simplest beginning point is to focus on the breath and notice the contents of the restless mind, returning mindfully to the breath after each mental distraction. A guided meditation is a good initial training vehicle. Stephen Levine's "A Simple Mindfulness Meditation: Focusing on the Breath and Noting"[2] is such a vehicle.

There are many other meditation practices, some of which will be explored in future classes.

As with Class 8 on Concentration, we begin with an *āsana* sequence designed to condition the body to sit comfortably for at least twenty minutes.

   I. *Āsana:* A Sequence for Sitting Comfortably
   II. *Prānāyāma*
  III. Concentration
  IV. Meditation
   V. Relaxation

Class 10
Deep Relaxation Techniques

Twenty-first century life becomes ever more stressful with the increased speed of communication, the compression of more work into less time through "multitask-ing," and the sheer struggle of most people to make ends meet financially. The singer is not exempt from these conditions. Even at the high school level, singers are over-scheduled with all sorts of activities, leaving little or no time for rest. The stresses on university voice majors increase as costs rise and students must work to pay them, and the young professional singer is pressed from all sides with demands that drain energy and raise the stress level. Without the safety valve of some form of deep relaxation, the nervous system is overloaded, and the singer's health is at risk.

Below the surface of the vicissitudes of daily life, however, there exists a deep state of balance. It is our natural state, and we can learn to tap into it at will. Encountering the silence and beauty of the natural world is one way that many people find this restoring feeling of balance. For others the entryway is prayer. If, however, there is little opportunity to be in Nature, or one has not developed a spiritual practice, there are relaxation techniques in yoga that "quiet the senses and lead us beneath the rest-less surface of the mind. Through relaxation we restore a sense of inner harmony."[3]

There are many approaches to deep relaxation, two of which are introduced in this class. The first, Progressive Tension and Release, can be done in a short period of time and almost anywhere one can lie down on the floor for a few minutes. The second, "31 or 61 Points," takes ten or twenty minutes and needs a place where one will not be disturbed.

   I. *Āsana:* A Basic Sequence Using a IN4/EX4 breath pattern
   II. Prānāyāma
  III. Humming
  IV. Concentration/Meditation
   V. Deep Relaxation Techniques

Class 11

A Practice for Diction

Unless young singers have studied French or German as languages or in art song with a good teacher, they are unlikely to have encountered vowel and consonant sounds that are significantly different from those in English. The eight sounds that singers must learn as soon as they sing in Italian, German, and French are the pure vowels [e] and [o], the rounded front vowels [y] [ʏ] [ø] and [oe], and the German front and back "ch" sounds [ç] and [x] (I leave the schwa [ə], which differs slightly from language to language, to the diction teacher.) For those lucky few whose ears are finely tuned and well coordinated with their articulators, the sounds are learned quickly. For most, it is a long process.

The technique of using sound in *āsana* is an excellent tool to aid learning to make these unfamiliar sounds. In each case, the crux of the matter is holding the tongue in an unusual position while making a sound. Avoiding the English diphthongs in [e] and [o] requires not moving the tongue, jaw, or lips for the duration of the vowel sound. Making the rounded front vowels is largely a matter of bringing the tongue into a forward position while keeping the lips rounded (or vice versa—rounding the lips over the correct tongue position). The German "ch" sounds require blowing air over a particular tongue position. In all these cases, using each sound as a chanting device while moving on the exhalation phase of repetition gives the student a measured practice in sustaining the sounds very much like singing. Attention will necessarily focus on maintaining the tongue, jaw, and lip position while moving the rest of the body.

It will be necessary to use a large easel tablet with the International Phonetic Alphabet symbols and a common spelling and sample word for each sound written large enough that the class can easily see it (one symbol per page). On the inhalation phase of the posture, the teacher chants the sound; on the exhalation phase, the students chant the sound. There are many creative possibilities for using this tool. The sequence in this class is a model that can be modified endlessly once it has been tried. In general, the two vowel sounds that make up a rounded front vowel sound are worked separately in a single posture and then repeated as the composite sound later in another posture. The "ch" sounds are chanted both as single sounds and in the context of a frequently sung one-syllable word. The sounds [u] [i] [ʊ] [ɪ] [ɔ] and [ɛ] are also used for forming the rounded front vowels.

The section of the class normally given over to humming various patterns uses these same vowel sounds for vocalizing long patterns. In this way, the student practices singing the sounds over a longer range and in various pitch patterns. Keeping the vowel sound true in these exercises further solidifies the student's grasp of the particular sound's formation.

It is important for the student to keep the tip of the tongue against the gum ridge, either just below the teeth or at the bottom of the ridge if the tongue is long, throughout the practice of each posture and each vocalization. Attention to this point allows the tongue to assume the correct position for each sound and, in addition, helps those students who tend to pull the tongue back during phonation.

I. *Āsana:* A Sequence for Foreign Language Vowel and Consonant Sounds
II. *Prāṇāyāma*
III. Sound: Vocalizing Vowel Sounds
IV. Concentration: Holding Sounds in Mind
V. Relaxation

Class 12
A Practice for Memorizing

Memorizing vocal music is a necessity for all singers, and there are various ways to do it. Some learn aurally while others learn visually. Among famous operatic singers, Kiri Te Kanawa apparently learned her roles by listening to recordings whereas Maria Callas felt that one could not look at the score too much. For some singers, memorizing music presents no particular problems; for others it is a struggle. Most fall somewhere in between, and there are always those students who wait until the last minute to memorize a song, not realizing that only sufficient repetition fixes the song in memory so that it stays there under performance stress. The use of sound in *āsana* not only benefits clarity and smoothness of tone, length of breath, focus of attention, elements of diction, and the ability to move and sing at the same time, but also can be used as a tool for memorizing songs.

The call-and-response (or listen-and-repeat) approach to learning and memorizing chants can be adapted to the process of memorizing a song. Coordinating the sound with movement into and out of postures makes use of the power of motion to reinforce memory. Extending the memorizing process to concentration and meditation practices offers the additional tools of visualization and embodiment.

Although using phrases of an actual song in *āsana* is considerably more complex than straightforward chants, it is workable with some practice. The song chosen for the demonstration of this process is Giordani's "Caro mio ben" for its more or less regular two-measure phrases and relative ease of singing. Even if most of the students in the class already know the song, it makes an effective demonstration of the practice.

After establishing at least a four-count inhalation and four-count exhalation in the warm-up postures, the teacher then sings the first phrase as the students inhale with the appropriate movements in the posture. On the exhalation, the students sing the phrase back with the appropriate movements. The inhalations and exhalations will necessarily vary according to each phrase length, though most are fairly consistent two-measure phrases. If four-measure phrases are used, the phases of the breath are greatly lengthened and movement is slowed by half. The repetitions indicated serve to strengthen the memory process. It may be desirable to use a metronome set at M.M. 60 for this practice.

After the *āsana* practice, a balancing and calming breathing practice prepares for concentration. Each student should choose his or her own song to be memorized for this part of the practice (and have the score at hand). The meditation practice on the meaning or emotion of the song adds depth to the memorization process.

   I. *Āsana:* A Sequence for Memorizing a Song: Postures with Singing
  II. *Prāṇāyāma* for Rest and Balance
 III. Concentration for Memorization
 IV. Meditation for Meaning
  V. Relaxation

Class 13
Review
A Complete Practice

By way of reviewing the elements of yoga practice that apply directly to the art of singing, this class will simply present a complete practice without teaching anything new. Beginning with *āsana* and ending with deep relaxation, the class will take the students through a complete practice of the type that can be done on a daily basis to enhance both good singing and good health.

It should be noted that the order of the postures can be reversed for a morning practice if the individual is very tired and needs to go from floor postures to standing postures to build energy. The number of postures can be varied, as can the number of repetitions and length of stay for each posture, to meet the individual's needs of the moment. Other breathing practices, as well as concentration and meditation practices, may be more suited to the needs of the moment. Relaxation can be normal or deep as needed. In short, this practice is a basic model upon which many variations are possible.

Humming may also come after Meditation or at the end of the practice as a way of bringing awareness back to the day ahead and warming up the voice in the process.

   I. *Āsana* with IN4/EX4
  II. *Prāṇāyāma*
 III. Humming
 IV. Concentration/Meditation
  V. Deep Relaxation

Class 14

Yoga and You

Exam (if required)

If this is a class for credit in the university system, an exam is probably required. If not, this last class of the series can serve as a way to get students to personalize what they have learned. The questions and exercises are designed to help the student think independently about a personal yoga practice and can be used as an exam or as a point of departure for future classes or personal practice.

Most of the questions and exercises call for totally individual responses. There are no right or wrong answers to those. The few factual questions concerning some fundamental principles of yoga call for straightforward answers and can form part of the basis for a grade if one is required.

  I. Basic Principles
    A. The Body
    B. The Breath
    C. The Mind
    D. Deep Relaxation
 II. Yoga and You
    A. The Body
    B. The Breath
    C. The Mind
    D. Relaxation

Second Semester with Special Topics

Class 1
Refining the Body

This second series of classes is designed to build on the techniques learned in the first series. All of the practices are presented in more advanced forms and many contain new material. The *āsana* sections, for example, contain approximately thirty new postures, introduced three or four at a time for the first nine or ten classes. Postures already learned will be practiced with longer stays, varied arm and leg adaptations, breath adaptations, and short *vinyasa* flows (three or four postures done consecutively with breath coordination) for ongoing physical development. Class 1 begins this process of refining the body. (Note: "Stay" occurs on the last repetition unless otherwise instructed.)

   I. *Āsana:* New Postures and Focusing on "Stay"
  II. *Prāṇāyāma*
 III. Concentration: Focusing on the Breath and Noting
 IV. Relaxation

Class 2
Lengthening the Breath

Both *āsana* and *prāṇāyāma* practices can be constructed to lengthen the breath as a whole or any of its parts. The singer, of course, is most interested in lengthening the exhalation part of the breath, as that is the carrier of tone. For those singers who do not use sufficient inhalation, practices that deepen the inhalation can develop the capacity to take in more breath. Suspension of the breath with the lungs full strengthens the muscles of inhalation and builds energy, while suspension of the breath with the lungs empty strengthens the muscles of exhalation and calms the nervous system.

The *āsana* section of this class works both inhalation and exhalation in various postures. Adding breath adaptations actually requires more physical work of the body and is an excellent tool for deepening postures and gaining overall strength. Because of the longer and more strenuous *prāṇāyāma* section, the *āsana* section is somewhat shorter to avoid fatigue.

The *prāṇāyāma* section is constructed to lengthen the overall breath cycle to a thirty-two second breath, a little less than two breaths per minute. This goal may not be appropriate for all class members at this time, but it is an excellent goal in general. Working up to a long breath is a gradual process and must be practiced daily. If at any time the student feels lightheaded, dizzy, nauseous, or too hot, he or she should stop immediately and resume at a shorter breath length when able.

   I. *Āsana:* Working with the Breath at Different Lengths
  II. *Prāṇāyāma:* Lengthening the Whole Breath to 32 Seconds
 III. Concentration Using "So-hum"
 IV. Relaxation
  V. Humming

Class 3

Singing in Motion

(and Unusual Positions)

Many of today's young singers have some experience singing while using patterned motions because of the prevalence of show choirs at the high school level. Singing while moving purposefully as a character, however, is a somewhat different proposition. This type of movement is more organically connected to the meaning of what is being sung rather than only to the rhythm of the music.

Young singers often have habits of movement while singing that have little to do with the music itself. Some are nervous habits; most are unconscious. In order to counteract these distracting movements, singers are taught to sing while standing still. Sometimes they feel that they are in a straitjacket and become quite tense. In fact, however, even standing relatively still there are micro-movements going on in the body that are natural to singing. Nevertheless, some singers, either through trying to stand still or because they are simply inhibited in their physical movements, have difficulty singing and moving at the same time.

This class explores the possibilities of singing while moving and of singing in unusual positions. Both motion and stillness in unusual positions are necessary for singers who will become characters on the opera or music theater stage. Practicing singing in yoga postures is a dynamic approach to freeing the body to move and the voice to sing at the same time. Because this *āsana* practice is quite complex and somewhat strenuous, the class will begin with *prāṇāyāma* to ground the breath and humming exercises to warm up the voice.

The three patriotic songs, "My Country, 'Tis of Thee," "America the Beautiful," and "The Star-Spangled Banner," were chosen for this practice because all the American students are likely to know them from memory. (If they do not, now is the time to learn them!) If this lesson plan is used in a different national setting, other appropriate songs should be used, depending on the common knowledge of the students.

Of the three, "My Country, 'Tis of Thee" presents the problem of an irregular number of measures, having only fourteen. This requires some juggling of breath patterns. The other two songs are regular in phrase structure and easily adaptable to the postures. Of the three, the National Anthem is the most like an aria, having wide intervals, high phrases, moving eighth notes, and a climactic high note.

The inhalation/exhalation patterns indicated are designed for a slow, full breath at the beginning of the song and then a shorter inhalation before each successive phrase. Since this practice will not involve the teacher's singing on the inhalation phase of the posture, a simple count will suffice.

   I. *Prāṇāyāma:* Grounding the Breath
  II. Humming: Warming Up the Voice
 III. *Āsana:* Movement with Singing
 IV. Concentration
  V. Relaxation

Class 4

Mindfulness: Being in the Present

Mindfulness, the quality of being present in the moment to whatever is in that moment, is increasingly rare and difficult to achieve in our frantic multitasking society; yet it is this quality that is necessary for creative work of all kinds. It is the quality that is recognized as "special" in communication on a personal level as well as in the communication that happens between singer and listener. In the singer it is called "presence."

Some people seem to have a natural quality of presence about them, while others struggle to remain focused. Regardless of natural temperament, mindfulness is a quality that can be developed and nurtured through regular practice in many different ways. This class offers practices for being present in motion and stillness, in the flow of the breath, in the sound of the hum of one's own voice, in a mental focus, in the heart, and to the whole self in deep relaxation. Being totally present in the motion of repetition in physical postures simulates being totally present in the motion of the music in a sung phrase. Being totally present in the stillness of "stay" simulates keeping the mind from wandering away from the music during interludes between vocal phrases or sections of a song. Slowing down the motion with a longer count increases both mindfulness and the amount of work being done by the body.

    I. *Āsana:* Being Present in Motion and Stillness
    II. *Prānayama:* Being Present in the Flow of the Breath
    III. Humming: Being Present in the Sound of the Hum
    IV. Concentration: Being Present to a Mental Focus
    V. Meditation: Being Present in the Heart
    VI. Relaxation: Being Present to the Whole Self

Class 5
Opening the Heart

There are always special people in our lives who seem to live through an open heart. For some, it is their very nature; for others, it may be the result of a catastrophic life experience. Most of us admire these openhearted people and wonder how we, too, can become openhearted.

    Singers who truly connect with their listeners on a profound level have this openhearted quality. Without this quality, the singing lacks the element of personal communication that so stirs the hearts of the listeners. Most singers want to sing in this way, but some are fearful of opening themselves too much in their singing. There are many reasons for this fear, most of which can be resolved with appropriate help. It is possible to reduce the fear and nurture the quality of openheartedness through practices that address the whole person in the context of the heart. Like everything else, achieving this goal requires constant practice. This class presents some specific practices to begin this journey.

    I. *Āsana:* Opening the Front of the Body
    II. *Prānāyāma:* Opening the Breath
    III. Humming: Centering the Voice in the Heart
    IV. Concentration: Centering the Mind in the Heart
    V. Meditation: Opening the Heart—"Loving Kindness Meditation" (*Metta*)
    VI. Relaxation: Opening the Whole Person

Class 6

Performance Anxiety

The term "performance anxiety" covers several different physical, emotional, and psychological states, some of which are normal and some of which are pathological results of deep seated fear. Pre-performance nervousness at the level of "butterflies in the stomach" is an entirely normal state without which the performer may not have the adrenaline level sufficient for an effective performance. If the butterflies are accompanied by extreme dryness in the mouth and throat, constricted breathing, and shaking in some part of the body, the performer is for some reason in a more heightened state of nervousness that is probably based in fear of something real (often lack of proper preparation) or imagined. If the performer feels a total lack of energy not related to fatigue, the problem can have a deeper psychological reason. If the performer simply cannot walk out onto the stage, it is time for serious psychological help.

In all of these states except the first (in which the performer is most likely eager to begin the performance), there are physical changes in body and breath that can sabotage a performance if not addressed beforehand. In the worst case, the singer probably should suspend performances until the underlying cause of extreme fear can be identified and worked through. In more moderate cases of nervousness, there are practices that can help control the loss of breathing ease and, over time, can help the singer release the old fears that produce anxiety. Even in the case of psychiatric help, a daily practice that includes breathing and meditation can be an excellent complement to medical treatment.

This class is structured to address confidence in the body and breath and to let the students explore their individual anxieties in concentration and meditation. If some students cannot do the concentration or become emotionally overwhelmed by what comes up, they should do whatever is best for them—sit quietly, lie down, or leave the class if necessary. Even these students should do the meditation "Letting Go into the Present" if possible.

   I. *Āsana:* Building Physical Confidence
  II. *Prāṇāyāma:* Building Confidence in the Breath
 III. Concentration: Quieting the Mind—Letting Go of Fears
 IV. Meditation: Letting Go into the Present Moment
  V. Relaxation: Synthesis

Class 7
Learning to Relax under Stress

Everyone has to learn to relax under stress for the preservation of good health, especially people engaged in public performance of any kind. Among musical performers, singers are the most susceptible to the effects of stress because the instrument is the body itself, and the power source—the breath—is the very thing often most affected. For this reason, it is necessary for singers to have some regular practice in the art of relaxation so that when stress occurs they know what to do.

This class is designed to lead to two techniques of deep relaxation that can be practiced on a regular basis. The *āsana* section is quite vigorous and includes Shoulderstand as well as a revolved seated posture. Contraindications for Shoulderstand should be observed for those students who should not do the posture.

   I. *Āsana:* A Vigorous Practice
  II. *Prānāyāma:* A Calming Breath
 III. Humming: Long Low Tones
  IV. Concentration/Meditation: "Big Sky"—Clearing the Mind
   V. Deep Relaxation: Finding Balance and Harmony

Class 8
Energy States

The average person generally tends toward one of three basic energy states: active, balanced, or passive. Stated another way, one is often either in a state of high energy, a state of balanced energy, or a state of low energy bordering on inertia. Yoga philosophy calls these states qualities of consciousness (*guṇas*) that produce different effects. The three are *rajas*, a quality of mobility that makes us energetic, active, and sometimes tense; *sattva*, a quality of illumination and purity that gives us clarity of perception and calmness of mind; and *tamas*, a quality of inertia and darkness that tends to prevent us from acting productively and seeing clearly. Not surprisingly, there are yoga practices to calm excess activity, energize inertia, and cultivate balance.

This class addresses each of these states with a short physical practice that includes both *āsana* and *prānāyāma*, a concentration/meditation practice that expands the mind away from personal concerns to an aware and inclusive state, and two relaxation techniques for different needs. It is useful to remember that in *āsana* practice, energy is increased with inhalation and backward bends and decreased with exhalation and forward bends.

I. *Āsana* and *Prāṇāyāma:* Three Short Practices for Different Energy States
   A. A Practice for Increasing Energy
   B. A Practice for Decreasing Excess Energy
   C. A Practice for Balancing Energy
II. Concentration/Meditation: "Big Mind"—Expanding the Mind
III. Relaxation

Class 9
Your Highest Value[4]

At various times during our lives it is useful and important to take stock of just where we are in the matter of living by our own highest standards. One of the most important of these times is in the late teens and early twenties, a time when most young singers are living in their first period of freedom from supervision by their parents or other authority figures. Although teachers, especially the private teachers, can be helpful at this time, there is no substitute for students having some idea of what their highest values in life are and a self-assessment of whether those values are reflected in their daily lives. This class is an exercise in that determination.

In his book, *Yoga for Transformation,* Gary Kraftsow has a wonderful practice for reflecting on one's highest value and on how much this value is present in daily activity, communication, and thought. It is a complex and rather long practice combining *āsana, prāṇāyāma,* and periods of meditative reflection on each of four questions. This class is based on Kraftsow's model but shortened, simplified, and structured somewhat differently, in keeping with the experience level of the students.

At the beginning of class, ask the students to identify to themselves their highest value in life, what is most important to them, and hold that in mind during the *āsana* practice.

I. *Āsana:* For Body, Speech, and Mind
   A. To Focus on the Body and Action
   B. To Focus on the Throat and Communication
   C. To Focus on the Mind and Thought
II. *Prāṇāyāma*/Meditation
   A. Your Highest Value . . .
   B. . . . in Your Activity of Body
   C. . . . in Your Communication and Speech
   D. . . . in Your Thought
   E. . . . in Your Daily Activity of Body, Speech, and Mind
III. Relaxation

Class 10
Changing Attitudes and Behavior

The first two limbs of classical Raja Yoga have to do with the moral principles that govern our relationships to others and the interior principles that govern our relationship to ourselves, and are the foundation upon which the whole system of practices rests. Attitudes are often rooted in the relationship to oneself, and behavior toward others flows from these attitudes. In yoga philosophy, the first limb (*yama*) consists of five principles of behavior toward others: abstaining from violence, falsehood, theft, extreme behavior, and greed. The second limb (*niyama*) consists of five principles of relationship to oneself: purity, contentment, self-discipline, study of scriptures, and worship of the Divine. These principles apply universally to all religious traditions.

All people who live long enough to walk and talk acquire habits of attitude and behavior that do not work well in life. In the maturing process, many of these are left behind as we form new and better habits. Some, however, that are rooted deep in our childhood experiences linger and disrupt our lives in various ways until we decide to change them. It is almost never just a matter of intention to change; there has to be a mechanism of change, the willingness to make a complete about-face, and some practice of mindfulness to keep us on track. One approach is suggested in the *Yoga Sutras,* Book II, Verses 33 and 34: "When harassed by doubt, cultivate the opposite mental attitude. Cultivating the opposite mental attitude is realizing that it is our own impatience, greed, anger, or aberration that leads us to think, provoke, and approve conflicting thoughts, such as violence. The intensity of such thoughts may be weak, medium, or strong, but their consequences, ever self-perpetuating, are always suffering and ignorance."[5]

Brain-imaging research is beginning to show just how the brain works in response to stimuli. There is evidence to suggest that enough repetition actually changes brain structure. This kind of evidence begins to reveal how meditation practices work to change the mind and heart of the person by changing the brain structure itself.

This class focuses on change: on doing familiar postures in a different way, on a breathing practice that helps to clear the mind for internal work, and on a different kind of meditation practice that works directly with changing a specific habit of thought or behavior.

   I. *Āsana:* Doing Things Differently
  II. *Prānāyāma:* Clearing the Mind
 III. Meditation: Alternating Focus for Change
 IV. Relaxation: Relaxing into Change

Class 11
Setting a Course[6]

At several points in adult life it is wise to check our direction in life, to make a conscious assessment of where we started, where we are now, and where we want to go from here. Perhaps the first of these points comes at some time during the years of higher education. Some students have a firm and workable idea for their direction in life, and some are uncertain or searching. Singers in particular need to have a clear idea of their direction, based on their gifts, their desires, and their means. Some lucky few can follow wherever a fine voice and natural abilities lead them; most need to have realistic options. This class presents a practice for self assessment of these questions.

A model for the span of life is the progression of the day from sunrise to midday to sunset. University students are still in sunrise but rapidly approaching the beginning of the long midday part of life, their productive years. Taking this model to simulate the passage of life, the *āsana* sequence takes the body and mind from Child's Pose through kneeling postures to vigorous standing postures and finally to prone and supine postures. The flow of breath and voice prepare for a meditation on the flow of life before relaxing into the flow of awareness.

I. *Āsana:* The Flow of the Body
II. *Prāṇāyāma:* The Flow of the Breath
III. Humming: The Flow of the Voice
IV. Meditation: The Flow of Life
V. Relaxation: The Flow of Awareness

Class 12
Constructing a Personal Practice

In yoga practice the ideal is to have a daily personal practice and attend class once or twice a week. The class provides instruction from a competent teacher, a time to learn new elements of practice, and a place to get any help one needs. It is just like the private voice lesson: one gets from the class what one brings to the class—aptitude, attention, and the work done since the last lesson. Yoga, like singing, builds upon itself a more and more complex, beautiful, and useful structure that both cultivates and reveals the inner person. Like singing, yoga invites attentive and loving practice. This class offers a basic guide to constructing a personal practice from the elements learned during this course.

I. Self-Assessment
II. Constructing a Practice
III. Obstacles and Commitment

Class 13
Review

By the end of this course, students should have some idea of whether the practice of yoga is good for them. The knowledge base of yoga is very large, and these classes have presented only the basic techniques applied to different topics. There will probably be questions from the class that will guide a review of these techniques. The most important connection to make is how each element of practice relates to singing and how an ongoing practice will continue to enhance their study and performance. This might also be a time to explore how yoga can be used in other performance areas; for example, in opera workshop, music theater, or stage movement classes.

Class 14
Exam or Self-Assessment

Notes

PREFACE

1. B. K. S. Iyengar, *Light on Yoga* (New York: Schocken Books, 1979), 13.
2. Iyengar, *Light on Yoga*, 11.
3. Jennifer Cook, "Not All Yoga Is Created Equal," *My Yoga Journal* (*Yoga Journal,* online edition, February 24, 2010).

CHAPTER 1

1. T. K. V. Desikachar, *The Heart of Yoga: Developing a Personal Practice.* rev. ed. (Rochester, VT: Inner Traditions International, 1999), 5–7.
2. Judith E. Carman, "Yoga and Singing: Natural Partners," *Journal of Singing* 60, no. 5 (May/June 2004): 8.

CHAPTER 2

1. Bernard Bouanchaud, *The Essence of Yoga: Reflections on the Yoga Sūtras of Patañjali* (Portland, OR: Rudra Press, 1997), 154.
2. Bouanchaud, *The Essence of Yoga,* 154.

CHAPTER 3

1. G. B. Lamperti, "Preventing the Decadence of the Art of Singing," in William Earl Brown, *Vocal Wisdom: Maxims of Giovanni Battista Lamperti* (1931; enlarged ed., New York: Arno Press, 1958), 5.
2. Henry Pleasants, *The Great Singers from the Dawn of Opera to Our Own Time* (New York: Simon and Schuster, 1970), 67.
3. Melissa Malde, "The Singer's Breath," in *What Every Singer Needs to Know about the Body,* with MaryJean Allen, and Kurt-Alexander Zeller (San Diego: Plural Publishing, 2009), 67.

4. Enrico Caruso and Luisa Tetrazzini, *Caruso and Tetrazzini on the Art of Singing* (1909: reprint, New York: Dover Publications, 1975), 13.

5. Goswami Kriyananda, *The Spiritual Science of Kriya Yoga,* 5th ed. (Chicago: Temple of Kriya Yoga, 1998), 223–224.

6. Jean Westerman Gregg, *From Song to Speech:* "Misconceptions about the Use of Humming as a Vocalise," *NATS Journal of Singing* 57, no. 5 (May/June 2001): 49–51.

7. Caruso and Tetrazzini, *Caruso and Tetrazzini on the Art of Singing,* 59.

8. Eddie Weitzberg and J. O. Lundberg, "Humming Greatly Increases Nasal Nitric Oxide," *American Journal of Respiratory Critical Care Medicine,* 166, no. 2 (July 2002): 144–145.

CHAPTER 4

1. Swami Prabhavananda and Christopher Isherwood, trans. and commentary, *How to Know God: The Yoga Aphorisms of Patañjali* (Hollywood, CA: Vedanta Press, 1983), 15.

2. Based on practices from Yongey Mingyur Rinpoche, with Eric Swanson, *The Joy of Living: Unlocking the Secret and Science of Happiness* (New York: Harmony Books, 2007), 138–145.

3. Based on practices from Yongey Mingyur Rinpoche, *The Joy of Living,* 138–145.

4. Based on a practice done in teacher training by Gary Kraftsow, American Viniyoga Institute Teacher Training (Austin, TX, 2006–2007).

CHAPTER 5

1. Eckhart Tolle, *The Power of Now: A Guide to Spiritual Enllightenment* (Novato, CA: New World Library, 1999), 19–20.

2. Gary Kraftsow, *Yoga for Transformation* (New York: Penguin Compass, 2002), 185.

3. Based on a practice from Lex Gillan, Yoga Institute (Houston, TX), Teacher Training Intensive (Ghost Ranch, NM, 1999).

4. Based on a practice in a Centering Prayer workshop with Thomas Keating (Houston, TX, 1986).

5. Based on a practice from Lex Gillan (1999).

6. Based on "A Guided Loving Kindness Meditation" in Stephen Levine, *Guided Meditations, Explorations and Healings* (New York: Anchor Books, 1991), 29–32.

PART II

1. Gary Kraftsow, *Yoga for Wellness: Healing with the Timeless Teachings of Viniyoga* (New York: Penguin Compass, 1999), 308.

2. Kraftsow, *Yoga for Wellness,* 309.

3. Kraftsow, *Yoga for Wellness*, 308.

4. Kraftsow, *Yoga for Wellness*, 309.

5. Kraftsow, *Yoga for Wellness*, 316.

6. Stephen Levine, *Guided Meditations*, 131–168.

APPENDIX

1. Sandra Anderson and Rolf Sovik, *Yoga: Mastering the Basics* (Honesdale, PA: Himalayan Institute Press, 2000), 197.

2. Stephen Levine, *Guided Meditations*, 90–94.

3. Anderson and Sovik, *Yoga*, 197.

4. Based on a practice from Gary Kraftsow, *Yoga for Transformation*, 191–214.

5. Bernard Bouanchaud, *The Essence of Yoga*, 116–117.

6. Based on a practice done in teacher training by Gary Kraftsow, American Viniyoga Institute Teacher Training (Austin, TX, 2006–2007).

Glossary of Sanskrit Terms with International Phonetic Alphabet Transcriptions for Pronunciation

Anuloma [ʌ nʊ ˈlo mʌ]. With the grain, specifically in the direction in which the hairs inside the nostrils grow (downward in the direction of exhalation).

Ardha [ˈʌrd hʌ]. Half.

Āsana [ˈa sʌ nʌ]. Derived from a root word meaning "to sit" or "to be present"; generally refers to the various physical postures of yoga.

Aṣṭāṅga [ʌʃ ˈtaŋ gʌ]. Eight limbs, referring to the eight parts of the practice of yoga according to Patañjali in the *Yoga Sūtras*.

Bandha [ˈbʌn dhʌ]. A muscular contraction, sometimes called a "lock."

Bhrāmarī [bhra mʌ ˈri]. A breathing technique in which a very light sound (like the humming of a black bee) is made on the exhalation.

Dhāraṇā [ˈdha rʌ na]. Mental concentration.

Dhyāna [ˈdhja nʌ]. Meditation.

Ekapāda [e kʌ ˈpa dʌ]. One-footed.

Guṇas [ˈgʊ nʌs]. Qualities of nature, i.e. energy, balance, and inertia.

Haṭha [ˈhʌt hʌ]. The yoga of physical postures.

Jālandhara [ˈdʒa lʌn dhʌ rʌ]. The *bandha* called "chin lock."

Kapālabhāti [kʌ pa lʌb ˈha tɪ]. A cleansing technique for the nostrils that uses a normal inhalation through both nostrils followed by a forceful exhalation powered by a strong abdominal upward thrust. This technique, sometimes called the "skull shining breath," also brings a feeling of energy and clarity to the mind.

Krama [ˈkrʌ mʌ]. Segmented, breathing or motion.

Metta [ˈmetː tʌ]. Meditation on loving kindness or compassion.

Mūla [ˈmu lʌ]. The *bandha* called "root lock."

Nāḍī Śodhana Prāṇāyāma [ˈna di - ˈʃod hʌ nʌ - ˈpra na ˈja mʌ]. Alternate nostril breathing technique.

Niyama [nɪ ˈjʌ mʌ]. Five principles of relationship to oneself.

Pārśva [ˈparʃ vʌ]. To the side.

Patañjali [pʌ ˈtʌn dʒʌ lɪ]. Yogi and grammarian who compiled the aphorisms of the *Yoga Sūtras*.

Prāṇāyāma [ˈpra na ˈja mʌ]. Breathing practices of yoga; expansion and control of vital energy as breath.

Prasārita [prʌ ˈsa rɪ tʌ]. Spread apart.

Pratiloma [prʌ tɪ ˈlo mʌ]. An alternate nostril breathing technique that alternates nostrils with throat, one side at a time.

Pratyāhāra [prʌt ja ˈha rʌ]. Withdrawal of the mind from the senses; the mental state that precedes concentration (*Dhāraṇā*).

Rajas [ˈrʌ dʒʌs]. A quality of nature characterized by energy.

Rajasic [rʌ ˈdʒʌ sɪk]. The mental, emotional, or physical state characterized by energy and action.

Samādhi [sʌ ˈmad hɪ]. Contemplation, or union of the individual with the universal.

Sattva [ˈsʌtːt vʌ]. A quality of nature characterized by clarity and balance.

Sattvic [ˈsʌtːt vɪk]. The mental, emotional, or physical state characterized by clarity and balance.

Śavayatra [ʃʌ vʌ ˈjʌ trʌ]. A relaxation technique called "traveling through the body" in which awareness is moved on the breath from point to point in the body.

Śītalī [ˈʃi tʌ li]. A breathing technique that uses the curled tongue for inhalation.

Supta [ˈsʊp tʌ]. Supine; on the back.

Sūtra [ˈsu trʌ]. A verse or aphorism of Patañjali's *Yoga Sutras*.

Tamas [ˈtʌ mʌs]. A quality of nature characterized by inertia.

Tamasic [tʌ ˈmʌ sɪk]. The mental, emotional, or physical state characterized by inertia and dullness.

Uddīyāna [ʊdː di ˈja nʌ]. The *bandha* called "abdominal lock."

Ujjāyī [ʊdː dʒa ˈji]. A breathing technique sometimes called "sound breathing" because of the sound made in the throat as air passes in and out.

Ūrdhva [ˈurd hvʌ]. Upward facing.

Utthita [ʊtːt ˈhɪ tʌ]. Standing; extended.

Viloma [vɪ ˈlo mʌ]. Against the grain, specifically in the opposite direction in which the hairs inside the nostrils grow, as in inhalation.

Viniyoga [vɪ nɪ ˈjo gʌ]. Mastering one step before proceeding to the next step in a process; the approach to yoga set forth in this book.

Viṅyāsa [vɪn ˈja sʌ]. Arranging or placing postures in a progressive order.

Yama [ˈjʌ mʌ]. Five principles of attitude and behavior toward others.

References

Anderson, Sandra, and Rolf Sovik. *Yoga: Mastering the Basics*. Honesdale, PA: Himalayan Institute Press, 2000.

Bouanchaud, Bernard. *The Essence of Yoga: Reflections on the Yoga Sūtras of Patañjali*. Portland, OR: Rudra Press, 1997.

Brown, William Earl. *Vocal Wisdom: Maxims of Giovanni Battista Lamperti*. 1931. Enlarged Edition, Supplement edited by Lillian Strongin. New York: Arno Press, 1957.

Carman, Judith E. "Yoga and Singing: Natural Partners." *Journal of Singing* 60, no. 5 (May/June 2004): 1–9.

Caruso, Enrico, and Luisa Tetrazzini. *Caruso and Tetrazzini on the Art of Singing*. Reprint. New York: Dover Publications, 1975.

Cook, Jennifer. "Not All Yoga Is Created Equal." *My Yoga Journal* (*Yoga Journal* online) (February 24, 2010).

Desikachar, T. K. V. *The Heart of Yoga: Developing a Personal Practice*. Rev. ed. Rochester, VT: Inner Traditions International, 1999.

Gregg, Jean Westerman. *From Song to Speech*: "Misconceptions about the Use of Humming as a Vocalise." *Journal of Singing* 57, no. 5 (May/June 2001): 49–51.

Iyengar, B. K. S. *Light on Yoga*. Rev. ed. New York: Schocken Books, 1979.

Keating, Thomas. *Intimacy with God*. New York: The Crossroad Publishing Company, 1994.

Kraftsow, Gary. *Yoga for Transformation: Ancient Teachings and Practices for Healing Body, Mind, and Heart*. New York: Penguin Compass, 2002.

Kraftsow, Gary. *Yoga for Wellness: Healing with the Timeless Teachings of Viniyoga*. New York: Penguin Compass, 1999.

Kriyananda, Goswami. *The Spiritual Science of Kriya Yoga*. 5th ed. Chicago: Temple of Kriya Yoga, 1998.

Levine, Stephen. *Guided Meditations, Explorations and Healings*. New York: Anchor Books, 1991.

Lidell, Lucy, with Narayani and Giris Rabinovitch. *The Sivananda Companion to Yoga.* New York: Simon and Schuster, 1983.

Long, Raymond A. *Scientific Keys Volume I: The Key Muscles of Hatha Yoga.* Illustrations by Chris Macivor. Bandha Yoga, 2005. Available at www.BandhaYoga.com.

Long, Raymond A. *Scientific Keys Volume II: The Key Poses of Hatha Yoga.* Illustrations by Chris Macivor. Bandha Yoga, 2008. Available at www.BandhaYoga.com.

Malde, Melissa, MaryJean Allen, and Kurt-Alexander Zeller. *What Every Singer Needs to Know about the Body.* San Diego: Plural Publishing, 2009.

Pleasants, Henry. *The Great Singers from the Dawn of Opera to Our Own Time.* New York: Simon and Schuster, 1970.

Prabhavananda, Swami, and Christopher Isherwood, trans. and commentary. *How to Know God: The Yoga Aphorisms of Patañjali.* Hollywood, CA: Vedanta Press, 1983.

Tolle, Eckhart. *The Power of Now: A Guide to Spiritual Enlightenment.* Novato, CA: New World Library, 1999.

Weitzberg, Eddie, and J. O. Lundberg. "Humming Greatly Increases Nasal Nitric Oxide." *American Journal of Respiratory Critical Care Medicine* 166, no. 2 (July 2002): 144–145.

Yongey Mingyur Rinpoche, with Eric Swanson. *The Joy of Living: Unlocking the Secret and Science of Happiness.* New York: Harmony Books, 2007.

Sanskrit Pronunciation Guide for Words in This Book Using International Phonetic Alphabet (IPA) Symbols*

Vowels	IPA	English Sound	Sanskrit Example
a	[ʌ]	as in but	*Krama*
ā	[a]	as in father	*Prāṇāyāma*
e	[e]	as in prey	*Eka*
i	[ɪ]	as in hit	*Viniyoga*
ī	[i]	as in bee	*Śītalī*
o	[o]	as in obey	*Yoga*
u	[ʊ]	as in foot	*Ujjāyī*
ū	[u]	as in moon	*Ūrdhva*
ṛ	[r]	as in saber (with a slight flip)	*Parivṛtti*

Consonants

b	[b]	as in be	*Bandha*
bh	[bh]	as in clubhouse	*Bhujaṅgāsana*
c	[tʃ]	as in church	*Cakravākāsana*
d	[d]	as in dental (tongue tip on teeth)	*Daṇḍāsana*
dh	[dh]	as in mudhole	*Dhanurāsana*
ḍ	[d]	as in ardent (tongue tip curled up)	*Tāḍāsana*
g	[g]	as in goat	*Guṇas*

Consonants

h	[h]	as in how	*Halāsana*
j	[dʒ]	as in juice	*Jānu*
k	[k]	as in kit	*Karaṇī*
kh	[kh]	as in sinkhole	*Sukhāsana*
l	[l]	as in trouble	*Viloma*
m	[m]	as in meet	*Mūla*
n	[n]	as in moon (dental)	*Nādi*
ṇ	[n]	as in trend (cerebral)	*Koṇāsana*
ñ	[n]	as in enjoy (palatal)	*Patañjali*
p	[p]	as in pit	*Prasārita*
r	[r]	as in red	*Rajasic*
s	[s]	as in sip	*Sattvic*
ś	[ʃ]	as in ship	*Śavāsana*
ṣ	[ʃ]	as in rush (tip of tongue up)	*Uṣṭrāsana*
t	[θ]	as in theater (very slight "th")	*Tāḍākamudrā*
th	[th]	as in courthouse	*Upaviṣṭha*
v	[v]	as in vat	*Viparīta*
y	[j]	as in your	*Dhyāna*

*The International Phonetic Alphabet is an alphabet of symbols of vowel and consonant *sounds* (as opposed to letters). The IPA can be applied to many languages and is commonly found in foreign language dictionaries and diction books for singing."

Note: The aspirate [h] that follows a consonant is a light expulsion of air following the consonant. Consonants with a dot under them are pronounced with the tongue curled up ("r" with a dot is a vowel sound and receives a slight flip). The difference between "a" and "ā" is one of length, though the IPA symbol [ç] approximates the sound of "a." The vowels "i" and "ī" and "u" and "ū" correspond to short and long sounds of the respective vowels.

Āsana (Posture) Index

Alphabetized by English and Sanskrit Names

([#] Indicates posture number from Numbered
Āsana List in Chapter 2)

English

Balanced Standing Posture (*Samasthiti*)
[1.], 16, 112, 201, 216, 221

Boat (*Nāvāsana*) [45.], 89, 112, 180

Bound Angle (*Baddha Koṇāsana*) [43.],
86, 114

Bow (*Dhanurāsana*) [29.], 68, 112, 180,
184, 187, 197, 199, 203

Bridge or Two-Footed Posture
(*Dvipāda Pīṭham*) [37.], 77, 113, 114,
118, 120, 177, 180, 182, 184, 187,
189, 201, 209

Camel (*Uṣṭrāsana*) [23.], 59, 203

Chair Posture (*Utkaṭāsana*) [6.], 26, 112,
177, 196, 208

Chariot or Airplane Posture
(*Vimānāsana*) [28.], 66, 112

Cobra (*Bhujaṅgāsana*) [25.], 62, 106,
112, 113, 120, 180, 184, 187, 192,
197, 199, 201, 203, 229, 231, 236

Corpse (*Śavāsana*) [34.], 74, 113, 197,
231, 233, 234

Downward Facing Dog (*Adho Mukha
Śvānāsana*) [18.], 49, 70, 113, 187,
196, 231

Easy Seated Posture (*Sukhāsana*) [41.],
83, 113, 114, 197, 201, 210, 211, 212,
214, 216, 217, 219, 220, 221, 222,
223, 225, 229, 231, 233, 234, 236

Easy Seated Twist (*Sukhāsana Parivṛtti*)
[49.], 96

Extended Lateral Angle (*Utthita
Pārśva Koṇāsana*) [11.], 36, 112,
113, 177, 196

Extended Triangle (*Utthita Trikoṇāsana*)
[10.], 34, 112, 114, 177, 189, 196

Eye Stretches [57.], 111, 114

Forward Bend (*Uttānāsana*) [3.], 20,
120, 123, 180, 187, 189, 192, 196,
208, 233

Half Forward Bend (*Ardha Uttānāsana*)
[4.], 22, 112, 180, 196

Half Intense Side Stretch (*Ardha
Pārśvottānāsana*) [8.], 30, 112,
180, 182, 196

Half Locust (*Ardha Śalabhāsana*) [27.],
65, 112, 113, 177, 180, 182, 187, 189,
197, 209, 231

Half Seated Twist (*Ardha
Matsyendrāsana*) [50.], 98,
114, 197

Head to Knee Posture (*Jānu Śirṣāsana*)
[47.], 93, 112, 114, 182, 197,
207, 209

Hero (*Vīrāsana*) [40.], 82, 110, 113

Intense Side Stretch (*Pārśvottānāsana*)
[7.], 28, 112, 120, 196, 207

Inverted Posture (*Viparīta Karaṇī*) [52.], 101, 201

Kneeling Forward Bend (*Vajrāsana*) [20.], 53, 113, 114, 119, 120, 121, 124, 177, 182, 184, 187, 192, 196, 199, 201, 203, 205, 207, 210, 229

Legs up the Wall Posture (*Viparīta Karaṇī, Supported Variation*) [53.], 103, 236

Lion (*Simhāsana*) [56.], 109, 114

Lizard (*Godhāpīṭham*) [22.], 57, 114, 184

Locust (*Śalabhāsana*) [26.], 63, 112, 113, 182, 189, 197

Mountain Posture (*Tāḍāsana*) [2.], 17, 112, 113, 114, 118, 119, 120, 121, 123, 124, 177, 180, 184, 187, 192, 196, 199, 203, 205, 207, 211, 212, 213, 215, 216, 219, 224, 229, 231, 233, 236

Mountain with Balance Variations (*Tāḍāsana with Balance Variations*) [13.], 40, 192

Neck Stretches [58.], 111, 114, 187

One-Footed Camel Variation (*Ekapāda Uṣṭrāsana*) [24.], 60, 207

One-Footed Forward Bend (*Ekapāda Uttānāsana*) [17.], 47, 192

One-Footed Pigeon King (*Ekapāda Rājakapotāsana*) [21.], 55, 114, 189

One-Footed Standing Big Toe Holding Posture (*Utthita Eka Pādāṅguṣṭhāsana*) [15.], 44, 192

Plough (*Halāsana*) [55.], 107, 113, 201

Revolved Head to Knee (*Jānu Śirṣ āsanaParivṛtti*) [51.], 100, 114

Revolved Triangle (*Trikoṇāsana Parivṛtti*) [12.], 38, 112, 114, 180, 189, 196, 205

Ruddy Goose with Child's Pose (*Cakravākāsana*) [19.], 51, 112, 118, 120, 121, 123, 180, 182, 184, 189, 192, 196, 199, 201, 203, 209, 219, 231, 233, 234, 236

Seated Forward Bend (*Paścimatānāsana*) [44.], 88, 113, 184, 197

Seated Triangle (*Upaviṣṭha Koṇāsana*) [46.], 91, 113, 114

Shoulderstand (*Sarvāṅgāsana*) [54.], 105, 112, 113, 201

Spread Feet Forward Bend (*Prasārita Pādottānāsana*) [5.], 24, 177, 189, 196

Stick or Staff Posture (*Daṇḍāsana*) [42.], 85, 113

Supine Abdominal Twist (*Jaṭhara Parivṛtti*) [39.], 80, 114, 118, 187, 197, 205, 231, 236

Supine Big Toe Holding Posture (*Supta Prasārita Pādāṅguṣṭhāsana*) [32.], 72, 113, 114, 189, 197, 236

Supine Bound Angle (*Supta Baddha Koṇāsana*) [35.], 75, 114, 189

Supine Forward Bend (*Apānāsana*) [36.], 76, 112, 117, 118, 120, 123, 124, 177, 180, 182, 187, 189, 192, 197, 201, 205, 207, 209, 219, 229, 231, 233, 236

Supine Hero (*Supta Vīrāsana*) [48.], 95, 113

Supine Lateral Bend (*Jaṭhara Parivṛtti, Lateral Variation*) [38.], 78, 114, 189, 207

Tank (*Tāḍākamudrā*) [33.], 73, 113

Tree (*Vṛkṣāsana*) [14.], 42, 192, 196, 207, 216

Upward Facing Dog (*Ūrdhva Mukha Śvānāsana*) [30.], 69, 113, 187, 196

Upward Feet Posture (*Ūrdhva Prasārita Pādāsana*) [31.], 71, 112, 177, 180, 184, 187, 231

Warrior (*Vīrabhadrāsana*) [9.], 32, 112, 113, 117, 118, 120, 121, 123, 124, 177, 180, 184, 187, 192, 196, 199, 201, 203, 207, 213, 215, 219, 224, 229, 231, 236

Warrior Balance Variation (*Vīrabhadrāsana, Balance Variation*) [16.], 45, 192

Āsana (Posture) Index

Alphabetized by English and Sanskrit Names

([#] Indicates posture number from Numbered *Āsana* List in Chapter 2)

Sanskrit

Adho Mukha Śvānāsana (Downward
Facing Dog) [18.], 49, 70, 113, 187,
196, 231

Apānāsana (Supine Forward Bend)
[36.], 76, 112, 117, 118, 120, 123,
124, 177, 180, 182, 187, 189, 192,
197, 201, 205, 207, 209, 219, 229,
231, 233, 236

Ardha Matsyendrāsana (Half Seated
Twist) [50.], 98, 114, 197

Ardha Pārśvottānāsana (Half Intense
Side Stretch) [8.], 30, 112, 180,
182, 196

Ardha Śalabhāsana (Half Locust) [27.],
65, 112, 113, 177, 180, 182, 187, 189,
197, 209, 231

Ardha Uttānāsana (Half Forward Bend)
[4.], 22, 112, 180, 196

Baddha Koṇāsana (Bound Angle) [43.],
86, 114

Bhujaṅgāsana (Cobra) [25.], 62, 106,
112, 113, 120, 180, 184, 187, 192,
197, 199, 201, 203, 229, 231, 236

Cakravākāsana (Ruddy Goose with
Child's Pose) [19.], 51, 112, 118, 120,
121, 123, 180, 182, 184, 189, 192,
196, 199, 201, 203, 209, 219, 231,
233, 234, 236

Daṇḍāsana (Stick or Staff Posture) [42.],
85, 113

Dhanurāsana (Bow) [29.], 68, 112, 180,
184, 187, 199, 203

Dvipāda Pīṭham (Bridge or Two-Footed
Posture) [37.], 77, 113, 114, 118,
120, 177, 180, 182, 184, 187, 189,
201, 209

Ekapāda Rājakapotāsana (One-Footed
Pigeon King) [21.], 55, 114, 189

Ekapāda Uṣṭrāsana (One-Footed Camel
Variation) [24.], 60, 207

Ekapāda Uttānāsana (One-Footed
Forward Bend) [17.], 47, 192

Godhāpīṭham (Lizard) [22.], 57,
114, 184

Halāsana (Plough) [55.], 107, 113, 201

Jānu Śirṣāsana (Head to Knee Posture)
[47.], 93, 112, 114, 182, 197, 207, 209

Jānu Śirṣāsana Parivṛtti (Revolved Head
to Knee) [51.], 100, 114

Jaṭhara Parivṛtti (Supine Abdominal
Twist) [39.], 80, 114, 118, 187, 197,
205, 231, 236

***Jaṭhara Parivṛtti*, Lateral Variation**
(Supine Lateral Bend) [38.], 78,
114, 189, 207

Nāvāsana (Boat) [45.], 89, 112, 180

Pārśvottānāsana (Intense Side Stretch) [7.], 28, 112, 120, 196, 207

Paścimatānāsana (Seated Forward Bend) [44.], 88, 113, 184, 197

Prasārita Pādottānāsana (Spread Feet Forward Bend) [5.], 24, 177, 189, 196

Śalabhāsana (Locust) [26.], 63, 112, 113, 182, 189, 197

Samasthiti (Balanced Standing Posture) [1.], 16, 112, 201, 216, 221

Sarvāṅgāsana (Shoulderstand) [54.], 105, 112, 113, 201

Śavāsana (Corpse) [34.], 74, 113, 197, 231, 233, 234

Simhāsana (Lion) [56.], 109, 114

Sukhāsana (Easy Seated Posture) [41.], 83, 113, 114, 197, 201, 210, 211, 212, 214, 216, 217, 219, 220, 221, 222, 223, 225, 229, 231, 233, 234, 236

Sukhāsana Parivṛtti (Easy Seated Twist) [49.], 96

Supta Baddha Koṇāsana (Supine Bound Angle) [35.], 75, 114, 189

Supta Prasārita Pādāṅguṣṭhāsana (Supine Big Toe Holding Posture) [32.], 72, 113, 114, 189, 197, 236

Supta Vīrāsana (Supine Hero) [48.], 95, 113

Tāḍākamudrā (Tank) [33.], 73, 113

Tāḍāsana (Mountain Posture) [2.], 17, 112, 113, 114, 118, 119, 120, 121, 123, 124, 177, 180, 184, 187, 192, 196, 199, 203, 205, 207, 211, 212, 213, 215, 216, 219, 224, 229, 231, 233, 236

Tāḍāsana with Balance Variations (Mountain with Balance Variations) [13.], 40, 192

Trikoṇāsana Parivṛtti (Revolved Triangle) [12.], 38, 112, 114, 180, 189, 196, 205

Upaviṣṭha Koṇāsana (Seated Triangle) [46.], 91, 113, 114

Ḍrdhva Mukha Śvānāsana (Upward Facing Dog) [30.], 69, 113, 187, 196

Ḍrdhva Prasārita Pādāsana (Upward Feet Posture) [31.], 71, 112, 177, 180, 184, 187, 231

Uṣṭrāsana (Camel) [23.], 59, 203

Utkaṭāsana (Chair Posture) [6.], 26, 112, 177, 196, 208

Uttānāsana (Forward Bend) [3.], 20, 120, 123, 180, 187, 189, 192, 196, 208, 233

Utthita Eka Pādāṅguṣṭhāsana (One-Footed Standing Big Toe Holding Posture) [15.], 44, 192

Utthita Pārśva Koṇāsana (Extended Lateral Angle) [11.], 36, 112, 113, 177, 196

Utthita Trikoṇāsana (Extended Triangle) [10.], 34, 112, 114, 177, 189, 196

Vajrāsana (Kneeling Forward Bend) [20.], 53, 113, 114, 119, 120, 121, 124, 177, 182, 184, 187, 192, 196, 199, 201, 203, 205, 207, 210, 229

Vimānāsana (Chariot or Airplane Posture) [28.], 66, 112

Viparīta Karaṇī (Inverted Posture) [52.], 101, 201

Viparīta Karaṇī, Supported Variation (Legs up the Wall Posture) [53.], 103, 236

Vīrabhadrāsana (Warrior) [9.], 32, 112, 113, 117, 118, 120, 121, 123, 124, 177, 180, 184, 187, 192, 196, 199, 201, 203, 207, 213, 215, 219, 224, 229, 231, 236

Vīrabhadrāsana, Balance Variation (Warrior, Balance Variation) [16.], 45, 192

Vīrāsana (Hero) [40.], 82, 110, 113

Vṛkṣāsana (Tree) [14.], 42, 192, 196, 207, 216

Index

Ananda Yoga, xv
Anusara Yoga, xv
āsanas. See Posture Index for individual
   postures
  arm movement as breath diagnostic
    tool, 14, 115
  cautionary note, 15
  chart for quick reference, 167–173
  for each area of the body, 112–114
    eyes and face, 114
    feet and legs, 112
    hips, 114
    lower abdominal muscles, 112
    lower back, 112–113
    shoulders and neck, 113
    spinal extension, 113
    upper back, 113
  general instructions, 14–15
  learning and practicing, 13
  positions and directions of, 15
  relation of tempo and motion to the
    sung phrase, 14
Ashtanga Vinyasa Yoga, xv
attitude(s), 161, 226, 240

balance, xv
  in diet and eating, 240–241
  equilibrium, state of, 148, 161
  in life, 6, 12
  physical, 160

in postures, 15, 16, 19, 20, 37, 40–41,
  42–47, 90
  sequence for, 190–192
  of temperament, 225–226
bandhas
  definition of, 136
  importance of, 136
  Jālandhara (chin lock), 136
  Mūla (root lock), 136
  a short practice for, 137
  Uddīyāna (abdominal lock), 136
behavior, 5, 6, 154, 161, 225, 227
being present in the moment, 239, 240
Bikram Yoga, xv
body, xiv, 3, 6, 8, 125, 127, 163
  as the acting instrument, 160
  grounded in, 115
  lack of awareness of, 10, 146
  relaxation of, 162
  singer's relationship to, 237–241
  as the singing instrument, 7, 10–12,
    159, 238
  as vehicle for living, 145, 164
  as vehicle of movement, 160
  of young singers, 4–5
brain, 7, 157
  alertness of, 127
  both sides of, 65
  of an opera singer, 146
  research, 154, 241

breath, 6, 7, 121
  in *āsana*, 14, 114
  breath adaptations in *āsana*
      krama, 115, 119–120
    metrical inhale/exhale, 114–115,
        117–118
    ratio, 116, 120–121
    sample sequences, 117–121
  as connector of mind and body, 4
  control of (short practices for)
    abdominal muscles pulled in too
        quickly
during phrase, 215
    abdominal muscles too tight on
        inhalation, 214
    breathy tone, 212
    insufficient inhalation, 211
    loss of breath during
        phrase, 213
    neck muscles tense during
        inhalation, 210
  development of, 8, 125–126
  directional flow of, 128
  as focal point for meditation and
      relaxation, 126, 144
  functions of, 127
  irregular patterns of, 115, 125, 127
  the singer's breath, 130
  in singing, 125–126
  in *viniyoga*, 10–14
breathing practices
  breath threshold, 131–132
  general instructions for, 128
  inhalation/exhalation, 128–130
  krama, 130–131
  ratio, 133–135
breathing techniques, 137–138
  alternate nostril, 138
  Anuloma Ujjāyī, 138
  Kapālabhāti, 142
  Nāḍī Śodhana, 140
  Pratiloma Ujjāyī, 140–141

  Śītalī, 141
  Viloma Ujjāyī, 139–140

Caruso, Enrico, 142
chanting, 7, 121
complete basic practice for daily use,
    193–197
  āsana, 193–197
  concentration/meditation, 197
  deep relaxation, 197
  prāṇāyāma, 197
  sequencing postures for, 196
concentration, 4–7, 12
  breath as focal point in, 126, 127, 144
  preliminary to meditation, 153, 155
concentration practices, 7, 148
  forming new habits, 150
  mental focus, 149
  setting a new direction, 150–151
  weakening and letting go of old
      habits, 149–150
contemplative prayer, 158

daily practice, 6, 148, 223, 225, 239, 241
Desicachar, T. K. V., 3, 11

"Eight Limbs" of yoga, 6
emotional states (*rajasic, sattvic,
    tamasic*), 103, 225–227
  anger, 223, 225–226
  anxiety, 225–227
  balance, 225–226
  depression, 225–227
  guidelines for assessment of, 226

Gillan, Lex, xiii
Gregg, Jean Westerman, 142

hatha yoga, xv
heart
  in meditation, 157–158
  openness of, 154

in singing, 3, 153
in yoga and singing, 4, 7, 8, 127
in understanding meaning, 152
humming, 7
  Bhrāmarī, 142
  as extension of *prāṇāyāma*, 142
  pianississimo hum, 142
  sequence for, 123
  and sinuses, 143
humming exercises
  arpeggios, 143
  chromatic intervals, 144
  long tones, 143
  major scale intervals, 143
  minor scale intervals, 143
  patterns and songs, 143, 144
  scales, 144
  three songs, 144
  wide intervals, 143

imbalance, 207
  in breathing, 125
  in emotions, 225–226
  in muscles, 207
sensory, 238
inner harmony, 3
inner self, 127, 154–155
inner silence, 153
Integral Yoga, xv
Integrative Yoga Therapy, xv
Iyengar, B. K. S., xiii, xiv, xvi, 6, 10
Iyengar Yoga, xv

Jivamukti Yoga, xv

Kapālabhāti, 142
Kraftsow, Gary, xiv, 153, 227
krama, 115, 130–131
  sequence for, 119
Kripalu Yoga, xv
Krishnamacharya, T., xiv
Kundalini Yoga, xv

Levine, Stephen, 239–240

meditation, xiii–xvi, 5, 6, 7
  breath as focal point in, 126, 127, 144
  definition of, 153
  and eating, 239–242
  for equilibrium, 161
  for influencing the personality, 153
  major effects of, 154
  posture for, 84
  practice of, 154
  process of several steps, 154
  role in alleviating performance
    anxiety, 153
  scientific evidence concerning, 154
meditation practices, 152, 155
  "Big Mind", 157
  "Big Sky", 156
  contemplative prayer, 158
  flowing river, 156–157
  focus on the breath, 155
  for memorizing, 225
  for mental blocks, 222
  Metta (loving kindness), 157–158
  for "presence", 220
  use of mantra, 155–156
memorizing music, 11, 161
  practices for, 218–219, 225
  sequence for, 124
Menuhin, Yehudi, xiii, xiv
mind, 3–8, 127
  and breath, 144
  and chanting, 121
  command of, 161
  coordination, instrument of, 146
  and *Kapālabhāti*, 142
  learning, instrument of, 147
  living, instrument for, 144, 145
  modes, 145
  one-pointedness, 146, 147, 148,
    156, 163
  of an operatic singer, 146

mind, (*Cont.*)
  and physical postures, 41, 43, 44, 46, 74
  relaxed, 148
  short practices for mental focus
    constant mental distractions, 217
    difficulty in memorizing music, 218
    lack of focus during lesson, 216
    loss of attention during
      performance, 216
  trained for performance, 148
mindfulness, 126, 145, 240–242
M.M. 14, 19, 115, 129, 133, 134
Muscles and joints of movement
  ankles and knees, 13, 175
  arms and shoulders, 13, 91, 95, 185
  eyes, 13, 111, 114
  feet and legs, 12, 13, 19, 112, 113, 175
  hips, 13, 34, 37, 114, 188
  neck, 12, 13, 81, 106, 111, 113, 114
    in *Jālandhra bandha*, 136
    sequence for jutting chin,
      200–201
    tension in, 204–205, 210, 235–236
    sequence to loosen, 185
    stretches for, 187
Muscles of breathing
  diaphragm, 126
  internal and external intercostals, 128
  internal and external obliques, 128
  palatal, 13, 128, 141
  rectus abdominus, 25, 126, 128, 131
Muscles of singing (postural), 12–13
  feet and legs, 112, 175
  lower abdominal, 2, 112, 136, 178, 180
  lower back, 12, 15, 112, 181
  pelvic floor, 12, 39, 87, 95, 130, 136
  shoulders and neck, 12, 113, 185
  spinal extension, 113
  upper back, 113, 183

niyama, 6
Numbered *Āsana* List, 15–111

Patañjali, xiv, 6, 11
performance anxiety, 8, 147, 153, 221
  short practices for
    extreme nervousness, 221
    loss of breath capacity, 223
    loss of energy, 224
    memory difficulties, 225
    mental blocks from early
      experience, 222
performer, the, 159
  communication with heart
    and soul, 161
  the whole singer
    the body, 159
    the breath, 160
    the mind, 161
    relaxation, 161
personality, 153, 227
Phoenix Rising Yoga, xv
posture and alignment, 5, 7, 159
  short practices for
    forward jutting chin, 200
    forward rolling shoulders, 202
    locked knees, 208
    neck, shoulder, and arm
      tension, 204
    slumped chest, 198
    swayed back, 209
    uneven stance, 206
Power Yoga, xv
prāṇāyāma
  definition of, 6
  presence in singing, 127, 146
    hallmark of great performers, 145
    short practice for, 219–220
principles of singing addressed in yoga
  practices, 7

Raja Yoga, xv, 8
ratio
  adaptation to musical phrase, 134
  definition of, 116, 133

effects of, 133
importance of, 133
relaxation, 5, 7, 161
  begins in the mind, 148
  deep relaxation practices
    awareness of light, 163
    short point-to-point
      awareness, 163
    tension and release, 162
    31 or 61 points, 162–163
    use of breath, 126, 144
  posture for, 74
repetition and stay, xvi, 12, 13, 33

sequences for specific areas of the body
  for balance, 190
  to loosen and strengthen neck and
    shoulders, 185
  to open and strengthen hips, 188
  to strengthen feet, legs, knees, and
    ankles, 175
  to strengthen lower abdominal
    muscles, 178
  to stretch and strengthen lower
    back, 181
  to stretch and strengthen upper
    back, 183
sequencing postures, 106, 196
Singers
  established professional, 6
  later years, 6
  opera, 3
  teens, 4
  university, 5
  young professional, 5
Sivananda Yoga, xv
"Skull Shining" breath, 142
sound in *āsana*
  description of, 121
  to learn something new, 122
  to memorize music, 121
  sample sequences

humming, 123
  learning or memorizing, 124
  vowel and consonant
    sounds, 123
  use of foreign vowel sounds, 122
  use of vowel sounds in repetition
    phase, 121
specific situations, short practices for
  after performance, 237
  after travel, 235
  before performance, 236
  excessive energy, 232
  extreme morning tiredness, 230
  low energy, 228
  restless mind, 233
spinal movement, 11, 128–129
stress, 5, 6
  in *āsanas. See* Numbered
    Āsana List
  breath under, 125–126,
    128–129, 133
  and illness, 226, 227
  in life, 149, 154, 237
  in performance, 161, 236
  relaxation under, 8, 163
Tetrazzini, Luisa, 131
Tibetan Yoga, xv
Viniyoga approach, xiv, 10, 13
  adaptation to individual
    needs, 11
  definition of, 11
  focus on function, 11
  goals of *āsana*, 12
  movement coordinated with metrical
    breath patterns, 11, 114
  movement of the spine, 11
  primacy of the breath, 11
  repetition and stay, 12
  use of sound in *āsana*, 11
Vinyasa krama Yoga, xvi
vocalises, vocalizing, 7, 11, 125,
    144, 145

weight issues
    chain of events: desire–intention–
        action, 240
    deprivation, 238, 241
    diet, dieting, 238, 241, 242
    eating, 237–241
        practice to change patterns, 241
    mental relationship to food, 240
    mindful eating, 239–241
    mindful eating practice, 240
    mindless eating, 237–239
    relationship
        between psyche and food, 238,
            239, 240
        to own body, 238, 240

yama, 6
yoga
    definitions of, xiv, 3
    lifelong practice, 6–7
    schools of in U.S., xv–xvi
yoga and singing
    classes for singers, 7–8
    connections between, 4
yoga for the private lesson. *See*
    Appendix
Yoga Sutras, 6, 11
yoga therapy, 227
Yongey Mingyur, Rinpoche, 154

Lightning Source UK Ltd.
Milton Keynes UK
UKHW011118200620
365252UK00013B/80